The Parent's Guide
to Food Allergies

The Parent's Guide to Food Allergies

CLEAR AND COMPLETE ADVICE FROM THE EXPERTS ON RAISING YOUR FOOD-ALLERGIC CHILD

Marianne S. Barber

with Maryanne Bartoszek Scott, M.D.,
and Elinor Greenberg, Ph.D.

FOREWORD BY HUGH A. SAMPSON, M.D.

AN OWL BOOK

HENRY HOLT AND COMPANY · NEW YORK

Henry Holt and Company, LLC
Publishers since 1866
115 West 18th Street
New York, New York 10011

Henry Holt® is a registered trademark of
Henry Holt and Company, LLC.

Library of Congress Cataloging-in-Publication Data

Barber, Marianne S.
    The parent's guide to food allergies: clear and complete advice from the
experts on raising your food-allergic child / Marianne S. Barber, with
Maryanne Bartoszek Scott and Elinor Greenberg; foreword by
Hugh A. Sampson.
        p.   cm.
    Includes index.
    ISBN 0-8050-6600-4 (pb.)
        1. Food allergy in children—Popular works.   I. Scott, Maryanne Bartoszek.
II. Greenberg, Elinor.   III. Title.

RJ386.5 .B37   2001   00-053920
618.92'975—dc21

First Edition 2001

Designed by Kelly S. Too
Illustrations by Betty Jean Flagg

Printed in the United States of America

5   7   9   10   8   6   4

For Lucas, who inspired me
For Virginia Barber, who believed in me
And for David and Helen Jaffe, who keep the commitment every day

CONTENTS

FOREWORD

Like all forms of allergic disease, food allergies have become more common in the last thirty years. Although at least 2 percent of the U.S. population, or about 6 million Americans, are believed to be allergic to at least one food, food allergies are far more frequent in children, affecting about 6 percent of children under the age of two. While the majority of children "outgrow" allergies to foods such as milk, egg, and soy, one of the most alarming trends in the past decade is the increasing number of severe allergic reactions (anaphylaxis) that in the vast majority of cases result from food allergies to peanuts and nuts. In fact, several studies have shown that anaphylaxis due to food allergy is the leading cause of severe allergic reactions treated in hospital emergency rooms.

To complicate matters further, we now live in such a busy world that fast food and processed foods—filled with the milk, eggs, wheat, peanuts, nuts, and soy that are responsible for so many allergic reactions—comprise the bulk of many a young child's diet. And anywhere you go, food is all around: it is the hub of virtually every social activity from birthday parties and school celebrations to a day at the ballpark, an afternoon at the movies, or even after-school soccer practice.

For parents of food-allergic children who know that just a small bite of the wrong food can spell big trouble, the vigilance must be constant:

every ingredients label must be carefully scrutinized; every activity must be carefully monitored. It can drive even the most reasonable families to distraction.

But now there is hope. For all parents of food-allergic children and all others who have a food-allergic child in their lives, Marianne Barber has come to your rescue with this authoritative, thoroughly user-friendly text. The mother of a food-allergic child herself and the survivor of many a skirmish on the food-allergy battlefield, she is no stranger to the anxiety and tribulation that seem to go with the territory. Writing under the guidance of both a board-certified allergist and a prominent psychologist, Ms. Barber gives readers a thorough description of the various food-allergic disorders and how to recognize them; how to provide a nutritionally balanced diet for the child who must eliminate key foods; how to deal with situations where hidden allergens may be lurking; and how to make appetizing food substitutions that will please even the most finicky eater. Her sections on marital tensions that may arise when different coping styles collide; interacting with your child's doctor, school, and relatives; and what to consider when traveling would benefit any parent dealing with a chronic disorder.

What's more, the book is a pleasure to read. Ms. Barber presents an incredible amount of useful information—from highly practical matters to the complex emotional issues that arise when dealing with a potentially life-threatening condition—in an engaging, conversational style. Then she seasons it all with a humor that can only come from having-been-there-and-done-that.

With an increasing awareness of how serious food allergies can be, many parents become depressed and overwhelmed when they hear their child's diagnosis. In the future I will suggest that they get a copy of this book, which will not only provide them with a wealth of valuable information but give them a whole new perspective on dealing with food allergies.

Hugh A. Sampson, M.D.
Kurt Hirschhorn Professor of Pediatrics and Biomedical Sciences
Chief, Pediatric Allergy and Immunology
Director, Jaffe Institute for Food Allergy
Mount Sinai School of Medicine
New York, New York

LUCAS'S STORY

It was Sunday afternoon, a steely cold day in February. The day after a punishing ice storm that had left cars strewn across Route 7 as haphazardly as an abandoned game of jacks. But inside, all was well. We had a good, crackling fire going and the Sunday New York Times *on the coffee table. Jazz played on the stereo. Our two boys were happily occupied. The house, for once, was meticulously neat.*

Bliss.

David, my husband, checked on our older son romping with a friend in the playroom, then wandered into the kitchen to make himself a peanut butter and jelly sandwich, as he'd done hundreds of times before.

But this time, our fourteen-month-old son, Lucas, begged for a bite as soon as he saw the sandwich on David's plate. "Eat?" he asked, blue eyes wide with hope, chubby body encased in red corduroy overalls, a buttery lock of still-uncut baby hair falling over his forehead. "Me eat!" he declared, reaching for the sandwich with a tiny, dimpled hand.

Well, why not? we thought, smiling down at him, so little and so determined. Let's give the kid a treat. We'd been cautious with him in the past—he'd had a bad bout of eczema as a baby—but this wonderfully lazy day seemed like just the right time to introduce him to our household's favorite food. Besides, it had just turned two o'clock. Lucas's snack time.

All it took was three tiny bites.

Within minutes, itchy little red dots appeared on the backs of Lucas's hands. Moments later, they were replaced by fat red welts that formed like bubbles before our eyes, boiling up to the surface of his skin and spreading outward. His eyes began to swell. His nose began to run. He started to cough and then to wheeze—a strained, phlegm-choked rasping. I unstrapped his overalls and lifted his shirt. The tender skin on his chest, now covered in welts, sucked in and out, in and out, defining his delicate ribs with each labored breath.

I looked at my watch. Just ten minutes had passed.

Hands shaking, I called the pediatrician, who called back immediately and said firmly, take that baby to the emergency room now. Willing myself to speak normally, I phoned my neighbor—"Sibyl, I have an emergency and I need you"—who ran straight over in her T-shirt to watch Dylan and his friend.

Coatless ourselves, we rushed Lucas into the car. Because of the ice storm the day before, the drive to Norwalk Hospital took fifteen minutes longer than usual, almost thirty-five minutes in all. David drove silently, steadily, carefully, concentrating on avoiding the slickest patches. I sat in the back next to my golden-haired baby, his blue eyes now wide with apprehension, singing him his favorite nursery rhymes. "Oh do you know the Muffin Man, the Muffin Man, the Muffin Man." He held his beloved Raggedy Andy close and tried to suck his thumb for comfort, but it was too hard to breathe. I held his other hand, completely red now but still so tiny and soft, and looked into his eyes as I sang, the best smile I could muster stamped on my face.

If he died, I thought, at least the last thing he would see would be his mommy smiling at him. At least the last thing he would hear would be his mommy singing to him. And then, of course, I would never smile or sing again.

Just a handful of cars had eased onto the road, fretfully picking their way around the streaks and pools of ice. Outside my window familiar landmarks came and went—the Caldor's where I bought the boys cheap pajamas and socks, the Shell Station that offered tiny race cars with your purchase, the new Toys R Us rising over the highway—but fear had pulled me deep underwater, the weight of it pinning my limbs and crushing my chest. Lucas's face floated above me, trusting and scared. I sang on and on. "Mary had a little lamb, little lamb, little lamb." Drive the damn car, I silently urged David. Drive, damn it.

By the time we got to the hospital, Lucas was bright red and swollen from head to toe. But still breathing, still alive. "Burn?" a worried nurse asked as we burst through the swinging doors. "Peanut reaction!" I shouted. Another nurse, slim and brunette, rushed us into an examining room and quickly listened to his chest as I eased his overalls down over his diaper. Narrowing her eyes, she raised her arm and gave him a quick jab of epinephrine in his pudgy upper thigh.

A miracle cure. The wheezing stopped; the hives shrank and melted away. Smiling now, the nurse handed Lucas a capful of Benadryl to drink, which he downed in a single gulp. Within minutes he was our peaches-and-cream baby again, breathing easily and cheerfully toddling about the examining room. I sat in the straight metal folding chair watching him, weak with relief, as David phoned the house.

We were lucky, the attending doctor said. Watch every bite he takes, cautioned the nurse.

My life changed on that day.

A story like this happens hundreds of times each day across the world.

Food allergies—from nagging skin or stomach problems to life-threatening reactions—aren't the end of the world. But there may come some days when you, as the parent of a food-allergic child, feel that they are. You may have days when you feel frustrated, misunderstood, isolated, confused, scared, angry, and depressed. Other days you may feel strong, optimistic, creative, powerful, knowledgeable, and resourceful. You will almost certainly feel stressed. It's all normal. As the mother of a young child who is highly allergic to peanuts, most legumes, soy, and fish—and was, until quite recently, also highly allergic to milk, eggs, corn, pea, tomato, and casein (a milk protein)—I've had all those feelings and more, sometimes all at once.

There were days when I could keep my sense of humor and perspective, and days when I could not. On the good days I could joke that my son thought Benadryl was a food group. I baked so many chocolate chip cookies to make up for the foods Lucas couldn't eat, I claimed that sugar was our staple food.

On hard days I would see parents all around me blithely handing their children peanut butter and jelly sandwiches, and almost shiver with fear. Every television commercial for peanut candy seemed like a personal affront. Every label seemed to read "may contain peanut frag-ments."

Now, three years down the road, it's gotten a lot easier for me. It will for you, too, even if your child's allergies or food sensitivities remain unchanged.

This book will help.

Writing under the expert guidance of a board-certified allergist, a prominent psychotherapist, and one of the world's leading researchers on food allergies, I have drawn on their breadth of knowledge and my own personal experience to create a complete food-allergy sourcebook that will answer your questions, address your concerns, and help you cope with the day-to-day aspects of raising a food-allergic child.

As all of us who have been dealing with food allergies know, those day-to-day aspects can be all-encompassing. Some tasks are fairly easy, such as learning how to organize your pantry or pack a safe and healthy lunch. Others are more difficult, such as learning how to decipher an ingredients label, making safe travel and restaurant arrangements, and creating special treats that get the kid seal of approval. And still others are truly challenging, such as handling emergencies, training caregivers and teachers how to handle emergencies when you're not available, and coping with the family tension that invariably accompanies having to deal with serious health issues on a regular basis.

One of the ways this book can help you right away is through its practical guidelines for elimination diets. An elimination diet—com-pletely removing one or several foods from a child's diet for a period of at least a week—is a relatively easy method for determining which food or foods are causing your child's allergic symptoms and is generally the first step all families must work through in the process of coping with food allergies.

Perhaps just the thought of a complete elimination diet makes you feel overwhelmed. Don't worry; we'll tell you what to look for and what to avoid at all costs. You may get eyestrain on that first trip to the gro-cery store (I will never understand why some manufacturers print their ingredients in white type on a black background), but once you've iden-tified your "safe" brands you're three-quarters of the way there. You'll have to read the ingredients every time to be careful, but ingredients don't change often and at least you'll have a starting point. We'll give you tips and special assistance in the following sections that will take all of the guesswork (and as much of the pain as possible) out of shopping and cooking for the milk-, egg-, soy-, wheat-, peanut-, and tree nut–allergic child.

This book will help you navigate every step of the way, from baking cupcakes that can pass muster with any four-year-old, to keeping your child safe away from home, to understanding why many marital conflicts arise around food-allergy issues and what to do about them. We give you in-depth information on the eight most common food allergies (milk, egg, peanut, nut, soy, wheat, fish, and shellfish), explain how a food allergy is diagnosed, and take you through the allergy-testing process. We have dozens of tips for avoiding the foods your child must steer clear of, nutrition charts that can help you keep your child's diet as balanced as possible, and wonderful recipes that incorporate "safe" foods into mouthwatering delights. We'll help you communicate better with your child's doctor, teachers, and caregivers. You'll find up-to-date information on the asthma, eczema, and environmental allergies (such as allergies to dust, pollen, animal dander, and mold) that affect up to half of all food-allergic children. And through it all, you'll learn how to incorporate living with food allergies into a safe, happy, healthy life for everyone in the family.

We're all on your side: those of us who've worked on this book, all the doctors and health professionals who work with allergic children and their families every day, and everyone in the Food Allergy Network, thousands of members strong.

As Anne Munoz-Furlong, founder of the Food Allergy Network, says in every newsletter, "We're all in this together." Please don't ever forget that.

The Parent's Guide
to Food Allergies

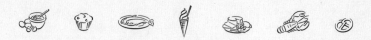

PART I

Eating

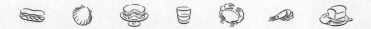

1

FOOD ALLERGY—A BASIC OVERVIEW

For many people, the realization that their child probably has a food allergy is a gradual process. Perhaps your baby was colicky long after most other babies had settled down, or had colic that came and went with no apparent rhyme or reason. Unexplained bouts of vomiting or diarrhea may have made your child miserable, like my friend Therese's son who was allergic to corn. Or your child may have had a chronic runny nose and bags under the eyes, like my friend Bobbie's son who was allergic to wheat. Many, though by no means all, children who are eventually diagnosed with food allergies suffered with eczema as babies and toddlers, like all of my friend Helen's children. Some, like my friend Bridget's kids, regularly broke out in hives. Others developed asthma, like my friend Jo-Ann's two boys.

In families like these, food allergies are a nagging health worry that comes and goes. Your child may exhibit no symptoms for days or even weeks at a time until suddenly one day the reaction returns full-blown. Or your child may always seem to be just slightly under the weather—stomach always a bit upset, nose always a bit runny, skin always a bit inflamed—not enough to trigger any real alarm but enough to cause justifiable concern. After all, how can you learn, play, and just plain enjoy being a kid when you're never feeling quite right?

For other parents, the first time a reaction occurs is an unforgettable event. For my friend Kate, it was the evening her two-year-old daughter touched a peanut and stopped breathing. For my friend Lisa, it was the afternoon she handed a Reese's Peanut Butter Cup to her restless toddler in his car seat, then struggled to keep her eyes on the road as he gagged and choked and fought for breath. For my friend Annie, it happened as she was nursing her infant son and he turned blue in her arms.

Even when the allergy is not life threatening, it threatens the *quality* of life for everyone in your family. At first, dealing with a child's food's allergies can feel a lot like being suddenly lost at 3 A.M. in a really bad part of town. Once you get used to things, it's more like the weekday commute: routine, but you still have to hit the brakes and veer off on the shoulder now and then.

So whether your child's symptoms are uncomfortable or truly severe, you are right to give them your full attention. Despite what your well-meaning friends or neighbors may say, food allergies are very real. And it is only by addressing all of the issues involved— from eating at home to traveling across the country—that we can keep our children protected and well fed.

WHAT EXACTLY IS A FOOD ALLERGY?

Although they may produce strikingly similar symptoms, there is a difference between an adverse food reaction and a true allergic response. So let's start with what a food allergy is *not*.

Probably the most common example of an adverse reaction is lactose intolerance. A child who is lactose intolerant is deficient in the lactase enzyme necessary to break down and digest the sugar lactose in milk. The intestinal cramps, bloating, diarrhea, and even vomiting that can ensue are guaranteed to make both of your lives miserable. If your child is lactose intolerant, you need to strenuously avoid dairy products or make sure your child has enzyme drops before eating them. But lactose intolerance is not an allergy.

A sensitivity to gluten (a protein found in many grains), which can be part of the intestinal disease known as celiac sprue, also has an extremely unpleasant intestinal reaction. It can make affected children feel awful or even become terribly ill whenever they eat foods such as wheat, oatmeal, barley, or rye. Needless to say, a gluten-sensitive child must be protected from gluten in any form. But gluten sensitivity is not an allergy.

Pharmacological food reactions are another form of food intolerance. In this case, the child is reacting to naturally occurring chemicals in the food rather than specific proteins. For children, the most common pharmacological reaction to a natural food chemical is a headache after eating chocolate. No, it's not the caffeine (caffeine can actually help headaches) but the natural food chemical phenylethylamine. This tidbit of information will be no comfort to your small chocolate addict, but at least it will give you some inkling of what's going on the next time he or she has a problem.

Finally, food additives and dyes can also, on rare occasions, cause adverse reactions. I found this out the hard way when my son Lucas began wheezing just seconds after starting to enthusiastically consume a yellow lollipop. The culprit in that case was tartrazine, also known as yellow dye #5. Other food additives that can cause trouble are monosodium glutamate (MSG), the preservatives known as BHA and BHT (found in many packaged cereals, cookies, and bread products), sulfites, and sodium benzoate. See page 136 for a quick rundown of which foods commonly contain these additives so you'll be better able to avoid them if necessary. If your child seems to react badly to any of these substances, you have but one option: avoid it. For the purposes of day-to-day life, whether or not it's an allergy is basically irrelevant.

A *true allergic reaction* is an immune system response. But instead of helping the body *fight* illness, which is how we usually think of the immune system's function, the reaction *creates* illness. That's because allergic people have inherited the kind of immune system that makes increased amounts of IgE, a type of antibody. When these people eat foods containing certain allergens—peanut protein, for example—the IgE reaction is set in motion.

When we all eat, whether we have food allergies or not, small amounts of food protein are rapidly circulated through our blood to our organs. If we do not have food allergies, or if we do but we're eating nonallergenic foods, the result is plain and simple nourishment. But when a food-allergic person eats an allergenic food, the IgE antibodies recognize the invader, and histamine-producing blood cells called mast cells and basophils become "activated."

Imagine a key slipping into a lock. That's how perfectly the antibodies and mast cells plus basophils fit together. And the moment that happens, the reaction begins. Almost immediately the mast cells release histamine and several other chemicals, and busily begin to make more. The allergy factory is up and running. And the food-allergic person is starting to feel sick.

The fact is, any of us who've had a cold or sneezed when the trees began to bud have experienced this type of reaction. It is the same combination of histamine plus other chemical products that gives us the sneezing, runny-nose, itchy-eye misery of colds and hay fever. That's why antihistamines are our first line of defense when it comes to treating cold and allergy symptoms. But food allergies are different in some crucial ways.

THE ANATOMY OF A FOOD-ALLERGIC REACTION

When a food-allergic child and an allergen-containing food meet, the child's histamine-producing mast cells go into overdrive. These mast cells are usually found where the body comes into contact with substances such as food, pollen, or animal dander from the outside world: namely, the skin, mucous membranes, lungs, and gastrointestinal tract. Wherever you can eat it, touch it, or breathe it in, you can have mast cells ready and waiting to react. So allergic reactions are generally characterized by hives (skin), swollen lips and tongue (mucous membranes), asthma (lungs), vomiting and diarrhea (gastrointestinal tract), or any combination of these symptoms.

Everyone has mast cells dispersed throughout his or her body, but different groups of mast cells are "activated" or "triggered" by different allergens. Some will respond to milk protein, for example, while others are primed to respond to pollen or animal dander. Some children have their reactions primarily in the skin and lungs. Others have most of theirs in their intestines. The only thing for certain is this: wherever the mast cells are triggered, that's where the allergic reaction will show up. So it is entirely possible for three different children, all allergic to peanuts, to react in three very different ways. One may have most of her mast cells triggered in her lungs and experience an asthma episode. The second may have most of her mast cells triggered in her skin and break out in hives. The third may have most of his mast cells triggered in his GI tract and throw up. They're all common reactions. The only thing that differs is where the largest number of mast cells are activated.

What's more, each food allergen has its own specific mast cell that seems to react only to that particular food. And those mast cells are not uniformly dispersed throughout the body. That's why children frequently react in different ways to different foods. A child who gets asthma from wheat, for instance, may break out in hives from eggs. The wheat-triggered mast cells are clustered primarily in his airway, while the egg-triggered mast cells are clustered primarily in his skin.

In the most severe situations, a child will have a food-allergic reaction in several different parts of the body at the same time. He or she may experience asthma plus severe hives, for example, or swelling of the throat, breathing difficulties, and lowered blood pressure. Whenever more than one body system is affected, the reaction is extremely severe, or breathing is compromised, doctors call the reaction anaphylaxis. Anaphylaxis is a potentially fatal condition. If your child has ever suffered an anaphylactic episode, you know how dramatic and frightening it can be. Immediate treatment, usually with epinephrine and an antihistamine such as Benadryl, is imperative. (For a detailed discussion about anaphylaxis and how to treat it, see chapter 2.) Thankfully, most allergic reactions are not that severe, although the number of children who have experienced anaphylaxis is on an alarming upswing.

WHICH FOODS CAUSE FOOD ALLERGIES?

Any food at all can cause an allergic reaction, but the following eight foods are responsible for 90 percent of all food allergies:

- Milk
- Eggs
- Peanuts
- Tree nuts, such as walnuts, almonds, pecans, etc.
- Soy
- Wheat
- Fish
- Shellfish

The allergens that trigger the reaction are specific proteins in the food. But even though a quick glance at this list confirms that the most highly allergenic foods are also high in protein, it's important to realize that even foods we don't think of as "protein foods" per se—potatoes, bananas, or melons, for example—do contain proteins that can cause a reaction from mild to severe in certain people. (Berries, widely thought to be a highly allergenic food, are actually ranked rather low in the allergic pantheon. Of course, some children are indeed very allergic to them.)

Unfortunately, four of the most highly allergic foods—milk, eggs, peanuts, and wheat—form the basis of many a young child's diet in this country. And soy, although hardly a major dietary component in Western cultures, can be found in many processed foods. In fact, the more prominent a food is in the food supply, the greater the chances are of people becoming allergic to it. In Japan rice allergy is surprisingly common. Seafood is a common allergy in Spain. In Scandinavia one of the most common allergies is to fish.

A GROWING CONCERN

Whether you are new to food allergies or have come to accept them as a fact of life, you have probably noticed that in the past few years you've been hearing about them more than ever before. There's a good reason for this: food allergy everywhere is on the rise.

Even if your child is not allergic to peanuts, you may have noticed that the incidence of peanut allergy has skyrocketed in recent years. This "peanut allergy epidemic" is not confined to the United States, although, like rock and roll, it started here first. We are, after all, a nation of peanut lovers. But as peanuts and peanut butter have been introduced into other cultures, the incidence of peanut allergy has been rising around the world.

Leading allergists have determined a direct link between how early a food is introduced and how common the allergy to that food becomes. As cases in point, both England and Australia have seen their rates of peanut allergy climb in recent years, from virtually non-existent to on a par with the U.S. incidence, as younger and younger children have been introduced to the joys of peanut butter sandwiches.

Here in the United States, where even young toddlers are exposed to a great variety of foods, it's not surprising that with their expanded palates comes an expanded allergy universe. Not too long ago, a Zwieback was as exciting as it got for a fourteen-month-old eager to exercise her chompers. Now, a "teething biscuit" can be anything from a sesame bagel to a cookie made with ground almonds.

Another theory that seeks to explain why there has been such a tremendous upswing in food allergy is the hygiene theory. As our culture has become more and more germ-phobic, we have come as close as humanly possible to sanitizing our young children's environments. There was a time when a pacifier that fell out of a baby's mouth onto a clean kitchen floor was casually popped right back in. Now, not only do we wash the pacifier in hot, soapy water, we wash our hands with antibacterial soap for good measure.

But new research has indicated something wonderful about the young immune system. It seems that we are born primed to ward off all the nasty little bacteria and viruses that have coexisted with humans for millennia. In fact, it's something we *need* to do to get our immune system in fighting trim. And if there's nothing for us to fight off, the immune system acts its age: like a bored-to-tears toddler in a neat-as-a-pin living room, it will all too often turn destructive. The result for an allergic child is an immune system so ready to attack that it sees milk, eggs, wheat, and the rest as the enemy.

Does that mean that we should give up and let the dishes pile up in the sink while dust bunnies collect under the beds? Of course not. Good hygiene is a crucial element in the good health and long lives so many of us enjoy. Certainly, the number of children who suffered illnesses and even died as a result of living in filthy surroundings is far greater than that of kids who now suffer from food allergies. But nature's lesson is clear: there's always a trade-off.

Standards of hygiene aside, some children are just genetically more prone to developing food allergies than others. If either side of a child's family has a history of allergies—*any* kind of allergies, including food allergies, eczema, asthma, hay fever, and allergies to dust mite, feather, and animal dander—it's probably best to assume that the child has inherited an immune system that's armed and ready to mount an allergic response.

But even given the predisposition for developing food allergies, it's not all out of our control. Children's immune systems, like their behavior, seem to respond best to clear-cut rules, enforced at as young an age as possible. If you are vigilant about never, ever, allowing your daughter to hit another child, for example ("The rule is no hitting!"), chances are that she will give up the hitting habit sooner than a child who is not so well patrolled.

The same often goes for allergic reactions. Children who strictly avoid a particular food seem to outgrow their allergy sooner than others. For many, though by no means all, children, age five seems to be the year when immune system responses are "locked in." If a child continues to eat a food that triggers allergic symptoms, whether vomiting and diarrhea, skin symptoms, or respiratory symptoms, the odds are no longer so good that the child will outgrow the allergy. This is because the immune system has not had the chance to "forget" the allergic response.

FINDING YOUR CHILD'S TRIGGER FOOD

Unless your child has had a severe reaction that could be definitely tied to one food (breaking out in major hives the first time he drank milk, for example, or wheezing after the first few bites of peanut butter), it can be challenging to determine which food in particular is causing your child's symptoms. The first step seems deceptively simple: observe your child. But like most tasks relating to children, this one isn't quite as easy as it seems. While it's common for food allergies to make themselves known within twenty minutes or so of eating, it's not unheard-of for an allergy to manifest itself a few hours later. Given the way that many kids graze, your child may have eaten three "snacks" in between ingesting the allergenic food and having a reaction to it.

Let's say your daughter, who is allergic to wheat, has half a bagel at 8 A.M., nibbles on some grapes at 9:30, enjoys a slice of cheese at 10:30, and then breaks out in hives at 10:45. Most moms would quickly conclude that the cheese caused the reaction. Maybe, but maybe not. The cheese may, indeed, be a factor in the reaction. Then again, it may have nothing to do with it at all.

To further complicate matters, some children will have a reaction to a raw food—apples, for example—but not to the cooked version. So don't necessarily rule out apples if apple slices are a problem but apple pie goes down with nary a hive or wheeze.

At this stage in the game, it's helpful to keep a food journal. Write down everything your child eats and drinks—and when. Note any reactions. Within a week or even sooner, you may have a pretty good sense of which food or foods are a problem. Now you're ready for the next step.

ELIMINATION DIETS

At this point, most doctors will suggest that parents try an elimination diet, centering on the food or foods that they think may be causing the child's reaction. You must completely and totally remove the offending food from your child's diet—not even a crumb!—for at least five to seven days to get any sort of accurate results. This will allow enough time for the reaction to subside—whether it be a rash from eczema, a reactive airway in an asthmatic child, or a chronic stomach problem. However, do not eliminate an important food such as milk or classes of foods such as milk, eggs, and wheat for more than two weeks unless instructed by your doctor. Little bodies need all the nutrition they can get!

The accompanying tables (© The Food Allergy Network) will help you optimize your child's daily intake while eliminating one or more common allergens from his or her diet:

STAYING HEALTHY WHILE ELIMINATING EGGS

IMPORTANT NUTRIENTS EGGS PROVIDE:	WHERE ELSE TO FIND THEM:
Biotin	Liver, soy flour, whole grain products
Folate	Liver, legumes, fruits, orange juice, green leafy vegetables (e.g., spinach, kale, and collards), whole grains, enriched cereals
Pantothenic acid	Meat, poultry, fish, whole grain products, legumes
Riboflavin (vitamin B_2)	Meat, poultry, fish, dairy products, green leafy vegetables
Selenium	Meat, seafood
Cyanocobalamin (vitamin B_{12})	Meat, fish, poultry, dairy products

STAYING HEALTHY WHILE ELIMINATING MILK

IMPORTANT NUTRIENTS MILK PROVIDES:	WHERE ELSE TO FIND THEM:
Calcium	Canned salmon and sardines with the bones, green leafy vegetables (e.g., spinach, kale, and collards), calcium-fortified soy milk and rice milk, calcium-fortified fruit juices
Pantothenic acid	Meat, eggs, poultry, fish, whole grain products, legumes
Phosphorus	Meat, eggs, poultry, fish, whole grain products
Riboflavin (vitamin B$_2$)	Meat, eggs, poultry, fish, green leafy vegetables
Vitamin A	Carrots and other bright-orange fruits and vegetables, green leafy vegetables, fish oils, liver
Cyanocobalamin (vitamin B$_{12}$)	Meat, eggs, poultry, fish
Vitamin D	Sunlight

STAYING HEALTHY WHILE ELIMINATING WHEAT

IMPORTANT NUTRIENTS WHEAT PROVIDES:	WHERE ELSE TO FIND THEM:
Chromium	Brewer's yeast; wheat-free whole grain products such as buckwheat, if allowed; liver
Folate	Fruits, orange juice, green leafy vegetables (e.g., spinach, kale, and collards), legumes, liver
Iron	Meat, eggs, poultry, fish, green leafy vegetables, cooking foods in a cast-iron skillet

Magnesium	Tree nuts, bananas, apples, peaches, lima beans, green leafy vegetables, seafood
Niacin (vitamin B₃)	Meat, poultry, fish
Phosphorus	Meat, eggs, poultry, fish, wheat-free whole grains such as buckwheat, if allowed
Potassium	Meat, poultry, fish, fruits (especially bananas), dairy products, vegetables

If you are committed to trying an elimination diet, the most important point to keep in mind is that it won't work unless you completely and totally eliminate as close to every molecule of the offending food as you can. Why so strict? Because even a trace of the offending food could very well trigger a reaction—and all your good intentions would be compromised in the process. For complete information on eliminating specific foods from your child's diet, see the chapters on specific foods that follow. You will learn, for example, that even if whey or casein (both "code" names for milk) is the very last ingredient on a box of crackers, you should not give your milk-allergic child the chance to have even one bite of that particular brand. What's more, you should avoid foods that are labeled *D.E.* (processed on dairy equipment, meaning production lines that are shared with dairy-containing products), even if the food itself does not contain milk or milk products. I know from personal experience that natural flavor, which can contain egg, milk, peanut, or wheat protein, is fully capable of triggering reactions in highly allergic little ones.

Elimination diets can seem like magic: you remove the problem food and *voila!* your child's eczema or wheezing or runny nose or stomach problems or hives disappear. You should be aware, however, that if you completely eliminate a food—egg, for example—and your child's allergic symptoms clear up, suddenly reintroducing just a small amount of that food can cause a severe reaction. In children with eczema, it may take just a tiny bite of scrambled egg to trigger a full-body rash; in children with asthma, it may take just some egg in ice cream to trigger a full-blown episode of wheezing. If you follow an elimination diet and your child becomes symptom-free, be sure to discuss your next step with your child's health care professional. Chances are, he or she will advise you to continue eliminating that food for at least a year.

If your child exhibits no symptoms in that time, you may have found your trigger. In all likelihood, eliminating milk and milk products from your child's diet will be the key to warding off such reactions. You may decide to visit an allergist to have the diagnosis confirmed. But happily, the odds are good that at some point you'll be able to reintroduce milk without ill effect.

On the other hand, you may find that despite your best efforts to completely eliminate a highly suspected allergen, your child is still having some sort of food reaction. It may be that your child wasn't allergic to the food you suspected but was experiencing a delayed reaction to another food. Or perhaps your child *was* allergic to the suspected food, but also to some other food or foods as well. So what do you do? You can keep on eliminating suspected triggers, one at a time. Look for the most common ones, like egg, peanut, soy, wheat, and fish. But the time has probably come to visit an allergist.

ALLERGY TESTING

Allergy testing is important if your child has experienced any of these symptoms after eating: hives, skin redness, itchiness, swelling of the lips or eyelids, throat tightness, wheezing, breathing trouble, coughing, vomiting, or diarrhea. Eczema may be the result of a food allergy, but not necessarily. And asthma is found with food allergies only about half of the time; more common triggers are viruses or environmental allergens such as dust, pollen, mold, or animal dander. Certainly, if your child has experienced more than one asthma episode, you should consult with an allergist to determine the cause. Allergists, of necessity, are asthma specialists as well.

But there's a good amount of preparation that needs to take place before that first office visit. It's important to assemble as much detailed information as possible about your child's medical history, eating habits, and other pertinent observations you have made. Did the reactions occur at home or in a restaurant? Do they happen every time or just occasionally? If you kept a food journal as part of an elimination diet, the information you collected is valuable. Also ask yourself the following questions: Have I moved recently? Carpeted the upstairs? Added a pet to the household? Has my child's diet changed significantly in the past few months? Is there a history of allergies in my family? Every detail you can come up with, no matter how minor it may seem, can help your allergist reach an accurate diagnosis.

If you and your allergist decide to pursue diagnostic testing, your child will most likely undergo one of the two most common tests for IgE-mediated food allergy: either the IgE radioallergosorbent (RAST) test, which is a blood test; or a skin test. You will be asked to refrain from giving your child antihistamines for a week before the skin test is performed. Antihistamines in your child's system would suppress the telltale histamine reaction, leading to false negative test results.

Neither of these tests is particularly painful, but of course blood has to be drawn for the RAST test—never a pleasurable experience—and many small scratches or pricks are made on the child's back for the skin test. Depending on how sensitive your child is, the skin test can be a fairly mild experience or a truly uncomfortable one. My son has usually found the yearly round of skin tests to be tolerable, but that may or may not be influenced by the fact that a special visit to the biggest toy store in town always comes immediately thereafter.

In general, allergists prefer to wait until a child is two years old to perform a skin test, for the results may not be as accurate in younger children. However, if your child is under two and has had some serious reactions, testing should be done immediately, whether through a skin test or the RAST test.

BLOOD TESTS

In RAST and CAP RAST testing one or more samples of blood are taken from your child, then sent to a laboratory. The blood is placed

---

RAST versus CAP RAST: What's the difference?

You may have heard some parents of food-allergic children talking about the RAST and CAP RAST tests, with a certain amount of heated debate about the merits of one over the other. But in truth, there isn't a major difference between them. Both RAST and CAP RAST tests are reliable radioallergosorbent blood tests that aid in the diagnosis of a suspected food allergy. CAP RAST is the brand name of the RAST test made by Pharmacia Corporation. When pressed to explain the difference between RAST and CAP RAST, however, many health professionals will say that they feel CAP RAST has a slight edge in terms of accuracy. But it is important to remember that any medical test is only as reliable as the lab that reads the findings. A clear and detailed history of your child's eating habits and possible allergic reactions is as important in reaching a diagnosis of food allergy as any tests performed.

---

on absorbent disks that contain specific food proteins. For example, if your child's allergic history seems to point to a peanut allergy, your allergist will probably instruct the lab to test for peanut, tree nuts, and possibly soy and other legumes, as these allergies are not uncommonly found together. Then the amount of IgE antibody produced in response to those specific foods is measured.

The units of measurement are called KUA/L. Each food has its own particular KUA/L "danger zone." For example, as reported by Scott Sicherer, M.D., in the April–May 1998 *Food Allergy News*, IgE antibody levels of over 6 KUA/L to egg, over 32 to milk, over 15 to peanut, and over 20 to codfish were "highly predictive (greater than 95% chance) of having some type of allergic reaction among highly allergic children." Dr. Sicherer does point out, however, that lower values, unless undetectable, "may still indicate a potential for having an allergic reaction." Especially in the case of the lower values, your allergist will take your child's specific medical history into account to make recommendations on continuing or eliminating certain foods.

SKIN TESTS

To prepare for a skin test, whether the method being used is a scratch or a skin prick, your allergist's office will assemble a tray of food extracts that correspond to the foods your child eats regularly, including the ones that may have caused trouble in the past. (Unfortunately, it's impossible to test for an allergy to a food that has never been eaten, as the body will not have developed any IgE antibodies to it.) If there has been a severe or anaphylactic reaction to any foods, your allergist may choose merely to place a drop of that particular food extract on the arm and not use a scratch or skin prick implement. In most other cases, skin tests are performed on the back. If there are many foods to be tested, your allergist or the nurse may even draw a checkerboard on your child's skin, delineating the spaces where each prick or scratch will go. In a skin prick test, the next step is to place a small drop of food extract within each square and prick the skin with a needle. A

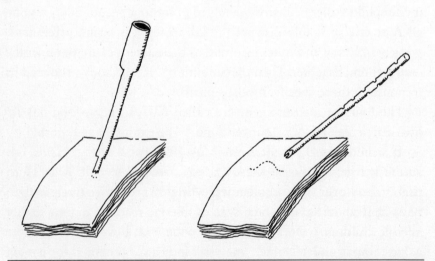

Skin tests are generally performed with one of two implements: the "scratcher" (left) or the "pricker" (right). Your child may experience some minor discomfort (mostly itchiness) during the test, but it goes away quickly.

Preparing Your Child for Allergy Testing

With any potentially scary or uncomfortable experience, most people, children included, do better with some warning. But warning too far ahead of time can just make a child unduly anxious. A two- or three-year-old might need to be warned about an allergy test only a few hours ahead of time, while an older child might do better with a few days' notice.

When you describe the test involved, whether it's a skin test or a blood test, be honest about what is going to happen. It may help to use a doll or stuffed toy as the "patient." Describe some of the sensations the "patient" is feeling, and express the "patient's" positive feelings, such as "I'm so glad we'll finally know why my skin is always itchy!" Reassure your child that you will be right there by his or her side through all the tests. And plan something fun to do immediately after, so both of you have something to look forward to!

scratch test uses a tiny, multipronged "scratcher" that has been soaked in the food extract.

A positive result to a skin test, indicating the presence of IgE antibodies, is a hive that looks like a mosquito bite. When describing a skin test reaction, allergists refer to both the wheal (the hive) and the flare (the red area surrounding the hive). It will appear within minutes and, like a mosquito bite, feel really itchy. A negative result—no IgE antibodies—is no hive at all.

It would be easy to assume that the bigger the hive, the more severe allergic reaction you can expect. Assume nothing. Remember, this is the world of food allergies, where strange things can and do happen all the time. The fact is that someone who develops a size 2+ hive in reaction to a certain food—the smallest size to be considered a reaction at all—can become extremely ill from just one bite, whereas someone with a big, whopping size 4 hive may have been eating the food for years and never felt any ill effects. What may account for the difference in the size of the hives is how many mast cells are triggered in the skin. Clearly, a child with mast cells triggered in the skin will not get as sick from a certain food as a child who has an abundance of mast cells triggered in the lungs or digestive tract.

Here's another factor that makes interpreting skin tests a true art: some food proteins—soy is notorious for this—will give a positive result on skin tests if your child is allergic to another food in the same family. That's because the allergenic proteins are extremely similar. It's not uncommon for a child with a peanut allergy to have a positive scratch test for pea and soy. Whether or not the child is truly allergic to the other two foods remains to be seen.

What's more, your child may have a positive skin test for a particular food, when in fact he or she is allergic to the nonfood member of its family: a positive test for melon, for example, when ragweed is really the culprit; or a positive reaction to rice or wheat, both members of the grass family, when in fact your child is allergic to the grass on your lawn. The proteins are very similar.

Happily, it is virtually unheard-of for a child to test negative for a given food and then have an allergic reaction after eating it. This does happen on occasion, but false positives are far more common. In fact, in the absence of any reported reactions, a positive skin test does not prove that the child has a true allergy to any particular food. If your daughter, for example, has been cheerfully eating peanut butter sandwiches three times a week for the past two years yet has a positive skin test for peanut, an allergist would tell you to continue feeding her peanut butter. In effect, she has been passing food challenges for peanut three times a week with flying colors, so there's nothing to fear.

So how *do* allergists accurately interpret skin tests?

The detailed in-depth, leave-no-stone-unturned medical history of your child that you prepared for your allergist is a vital piece in the puzzle. Let's say your son's scratch test was positive for soy and peanut, but he happily and healthily drank a soy-based formula throughout infancy and toddlerhood; what should you make of that soy reaction? You and your allergist will decide. On the other hand, if your son's reaction to shrimp was minimal—a size 2+, let's say— your allergist might still advise you to keep him from taking even a

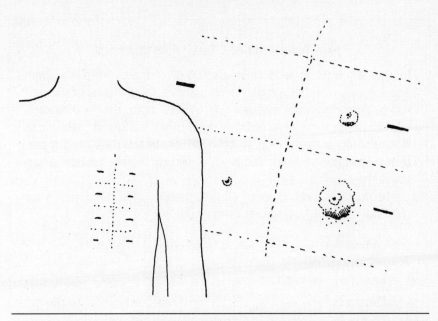

A negative skin test looks like a small red dot (top left). A positive skin test may range from a small hive or blotch to a very large one (bottom right).

bite of shrimp or lobster, as shellfish is such a highly allergenic substance, capable of quickly producing a life-threatening reaction.

There are times when an allergist will call for a skin test and a RAST test to be used in conjunction, particularly when the child appears to be sensitive to a variety of foods, but there are no clear indicators as to which. If both the skin and RAST tests come back positive for any given food, the diagnosis is clear. But it doesn't always work out that way. When the skin test is positive (as many skin tests are, regardless of whether or not a true allergy exists) but the RAST is indeterminate, and there doesn't seem to be a clear history of a problem, there is only one way to get to the heart of the matter: by conducting a food challenge in a hospital setting.

Although they don't occur very often, there are a couple of other situations that call for a food challenge as well: a child may be brought in for allergy testing, given the standard scratch tests, and test positive for . . . virtually everything. When a RAST test is

Skin Tests and RAST Tests: Pros and Cons

Neither skin tests nor blood tests are 100 percent accurate all the time. The accuracy of either is highly dependent on the skill level of the person performing and/or evaluating it. What's more, the food extracts used to perform the tests can vary significantly in strength, which can lead to different results. Overall, however, allergy testing is a highly predictive indicator of which foods your child can safely eat and which should be avoided.

The following points will help you better understand why your child's allergist may be making certain choices.

Skin Test: Pro
- Not very invasive
- Results are available right away
- Highly accurate; false negatives are rare

Skin Test: Con
- Not a good choice for a child with a strong history of anaphylaxis. (Some allergists will put a small drop of extract on the surface of the child's skin rather than scratching the skin in these cases.)
- Not as finely detailed a reading as a blood test
- Strength of extract may vary
- Child must stay off antihistamines for seven days prior

RAST Test: Pro
- Highly accurate; provides detailed information
- When performed every few years, it may give an indication of whether the child's antibody values are dropping

RAST Test: Con
- Blood must be drawn
- Only as reliable as the lab that performs the test

performed, the results are similar. Or the child may test positive to so many key foods—let's say milk, egg, wheat, corn, beef, and chicken—that it would be very hard to create a balanced, nutritious diet that the child would actually eat. Clearly no child, unless absolutely necessary, should have to subsist on such a limited selection of foods.

Preparing for a Food Challenge

Food challenges make for a pretty long—and tense—day in a hospital room, so it's best to pack accordingly. Depending on your child's age, coloring books, sticker books, small toys, favorite tapes and video games, and a beloved stuffed friend will all be welcome to make the time pass more quickly.

In most cases you will be asked to report to the hospital early in the morning so that the challenge can be performed on an empty stomach. (Food in the stomach may delay the absorption of the food being challenged.) It is best that your child have nothing but sips of water for at least two hours prior to the challenge.

Your child will probably need to have an intravenous access device called a heparin-lock inserted before the challenge. Yes, it is inserted into a vein in your child's arm—never fun—but it is an important safety precaution. Epinephrine and Benadryl are always prepared and on hand for your child.

The challenge food will be fed to your child in very small doses at fifteen-minute intervals. Your child will be closely observed at all times. If there are signs of a reaction, the challenge is stopped and the reaction is treated immediately. It takes about an hour and fifteen minutes to complete each portion of the challenge.

If your child completes the double-blind challenge without a reaction, an open challenge to that food will follow. If peanut was the suspected allergen, for example, your child may be fed peanut butter on crackers. The point is to have the child *know* what food he or she is eating, and not have a reaction—physical or psychological—to the experience.

But running the risk of a serious allergic reaction is definitely out of the question as well.

THE DOUBLE-BLIND PLACEBO-CONTROLLED FOOD CHALLENGE

Only one test can determine a child's allergies once and for all. Both the gold standard for allergy testing and the test of last resort, it is a procedure that must be performed in a hospital setting. In essence, it consists of feeding a child small quantities of foods—not only foods the child may be allergic to, but also foods that he or she is definitely not allergic to—under strictly controlled conditions. It is called the Double-Blind Placebo-Controlled Food Challenge (DBPCFC).

What does the name mean?

Double-blind means that neither the child, nor the health care professional who is feeding the child, knows what suspected allergen, if any, is being offered at each "taste test." (Of course, the dieticians preparing the tests know. Each sample is carefully coded and tracked.) The reason for a test to be performed on a double-blind basis is to rule out any psychological reactions. For example, a boy who is told that he is being challenged with egg, but fears that he is extremely allergic to that food, may very well show symptoms such as asthma, vomiting, or diarrhea. The problem is, those symptoms may just as well come from anxiety and not represent an immune system response.

Similarly, if the health care worker feeding the boy knows that she is giving him an allergenic substance, she may very well feel a bit anxious herself. There's a chance that she will indirectly communicate that anxiety to the boy through her body language and tone of voice. Frequently, before a DBPCFC is performed on a child, the dietician preparing the test will call the child's parents and ask about food preferences so that the food to be tested can be "hidden" in a favorite food.

Placebo-controlled means that not every "taste test" contains an allergenic substance. Sometimes it contains a placebo—a harmless nonallergenic food substance. Again, the placebo-control helps differentiate between true allergic reactions and psychological ones. A child who complains of nausea or other symptoms after ingesting a placebo is most likely reacting to the *idea* of the test, rather than the test itself.

It is important to compare the reaction to the placebo with the reaction to the actual food. If a child complains of the same degree of nausea or other symptoms both times, and the health care professional's observations of the child are the same both times, chances are that the child can indeed eat the food safely but is feeling a lot of anxiety about the test. (Clearly, placebo-controls are easier to scientifically evaluate with infants and young toddlers, who don't have a clue as to what's actually going on.)

A *food challenge* is simply offering a possible allergen to a child: a half teaspoon of yogurt to a girl who may be allergic to milk, or half a cashew to a boy who may be allergic to tree nuts. Literally, the challenge is to the child's immune system; it is just as much a challenge to a parent's nerve. Food challenges are risky. You should never undertake a food challenge at home without your allergist's approval if you know or strongly suspect that your child is allergic to the food in question.

When skin tests indicate that your child has outgrown some allergies, your allergist may ask you to challenge your child with those foods. The allergist will tell you exactly what the quantities of food should be and how many times a day you should offer the food to your child. In that case, there's little need to worry. Stick to the rules and you'll be OK.

Put simply, a Double-Blind Placebo-Controlled Food Challenge involves checking your child into a hospital for a specified length of stay. During that time, your child will be fed suspected allergens disguised in other foods, in order to determine once and for all which foods can be tolerated and which ones cannot.

When a child responds well to a blind challenge, an open challenge is usually performed. In an open food challenge, your child will be given a "normal serving" of a particular food, which is not hidden in any way. When your child has successfully completed this stage of testing, you can rule out an allergy to that food.

While he was at the Johns Hopkins University of Medicine in Baltimore, Dr. Hugh A. Sampson and Deborah G. Ho (also of Johns Hopkins) wrote about a DBPCFC they developed and directed. Their findings were published in the October 1997 issue of the *Journal of Allergy and Clinical Immunology*. In the article, they describe a ten-year study evaluating 300 children and adolescents for food hypersensitivity by use of the DBPCFC. These young people had already had positive skin test results to a variety of foods. In this particular group, egg, milk, and peanut accounted for 85 percent of the severe reactions described. The study was careful to include children with wheat and soy allergy as well.

The DBPCFC was performed by offering the child up to ten grams of dehydrated food—camouflaged in juice, infant formula, or moist food such as cream of rice cereal—over a ninety-minute period. Each child underwent two challenges, separated by about four hours, in a given day. One challenge contained the suspected allergen, while the other contained a placebo. Challenges were not performed when the child had clearly experienced a severe allergic reaction to the food, which was confirmed by a positive skin test.

During the course of the DBPCFC, if a child had a reaction to the allergen, symptoms developed within minutes to two hours of the food challenge. Overall, most children reacted to three or fewer foods. Those children who did not react to a suspected allergen were openly challenged with a sizable quantity of the food.

Interestingly, this study group also had a high rate of environmental allergies, particularly to dust mites, cats, and dogs.

What Dr. Sampson and Ms. Ho established in their research was that skin testing for these children was far more accurate for predicting the *absence* of a food allergy (over 95 percent accuracy) than it was for predicting the *presence* of a food allergy (less than 50 percent accuracy).

What we, as parents, can take away from that is a genuine sense of confidence that no allergy "bogeymen" are going to rear their ugly heads at us out of nowhere. If your child tests negative to certain foods he or she has eaten in the past—even foods you may consider to be highly allergenic, such as fish or nuts—you can rest assured that your child can safely eat them.

Clearly the DBPCFC is the test of last resort. But if you happen to be the parent of a child who needs it, it will give you definite answers. And as we all know, the more information we have, the better we can build healthy, safe, enjoyable lives for our families.

NUTRITION AND FOOD ALLERGY

Once you know what your child is allergic to, you can figure out what foods to avoid and what foods to serve without guilt or fear. Many children with food allergies can eat a perfectly healthy, tasty, well-balanced diet by simply omitting their trigger food. Nobody *needs* to eat peanuts, tree nuts, eggs, shellfish, or fish to stay healthy, and in fact lots of children don't eat these foods anyway, simply because they don't like them. But if many foods must be eliminated, or if a key food group such as dairy is taboo, it's important to take a good look at the big picture and be sure your child is getting the proper nutrition.

You can start by studying the tables that follow. (These tables are reproduced with the permission of the Elliot and Roslyn Jaffe Institute for Food Allergy at Mount Sinai Medical Center.) They will help you determine if your child's allergen-free diet may affect his or her nutritional status on a long-term basis. Certain nutrients are readily available in many foods. Others, no less important, are trickier to work into a daily routine.

VITAMIN GUIDE

VITAMIN NAME	CHIEF FUNCTION IN THE BODY	SIGNIFICANT SOURCES
A	Visual adaptation to light and dark; growth of skin and mucous membrane	Retinol (animal foods): liver, egg yolk, fortified milk, cheese, cream, butter, and fortified margarine
D	Absorption of calcium and phosphorus; calcification of bones	Self-synthesis from sunlight; fortified milk, fortified margarine, eggs, liver, and fish oils

E	Antioxidant, stabilization of cell membrane, protection of polyunsaturated fatty acids and vitamin A	Polyunsaturated plant oils, green leafy vegetables, wheat germ, whole grain products, nuts, and seeds
K	Normal blood clotting	Bacterial synthesis in the digestive tract; green leafy vegetables, milk and dairy products, meats, eggs, and cereals
Thiamin (B_1)	Coenzyme in carbohydrate metabolism; normal function of the heart, nerves, and muscle	Pork, beef, liver, whole or enriched grains, legumes, and nuts
Riboflavin (B_2)	Coenzyme in protein and energy metabolism	Milk, yogurt, cottage cheese, meat, green leafy vegetables, whole or enriched grains, and cereals
Niacin (B_3)	Coenzyme in energy production; health of skin; normal function of stomach, intestines, and nervous system	Meat, peanuts, legumes, and whole or enriched grains
Pyridoxine (B_6)	Coenzyme in amino acid metabolism; conversion of tryptophan to niacin; synthesis of red blood cell in hemoglobin	Grains, seeds, liver, meats, milk, eggs, and vegetables
Cyanocobalamin (B_{12})	Coenzyme in synthesis of red blood cells in hemoglobin (which carries oxygen in the blood); formation of blood cells	Animal products: meat, fish, poultry, shellfish, milk, cheese, and eggs

Folate acid	Part of DNA; growth and development of red blood cells	Liver, green leafy vegetables, legumes, seeds, and yeast
Pantothenic acid	Part of coenzyme A, which is used in energy metabolism; formation of fat, cholesterol, and heme; activation of amino acids	Meats, cereals, legumes, milk, fruits, and vegetables
Biotin	Part of coenzyme A, which is used in energy metabolism; involved in lipid synthesis, amino acid metabolism, and glycogen synthesis	Liver, egg yolk, soy flour, cereals, tomatoes, and yeast
C	Collagen synthesis (strengthens blood vessel walls, forms scar tissue, encourages bone growth); antioxidant; thyroxine synthesis; strengthens resistance to infection; helps with absorption of iron	Citrus fruits, tomato, cabbage, green leafy vegetables, potatoes, peppers, cantaloupe, strawberries, melons, papayas, and mangos

MINERAL AND TRACE ELEMENT GUIDE

MINERAL NAME	CHIEF FUNCTIONS IN THE BODY	SIGNIFICANT SOURCES
Calcium	Bone and teeth formation; involved in normal muscle contraction and relaxation, nerve functioning, blood clotting, and blood pressure	Milk and milk products, small fish with bones, green leafy vegetables, legumes, calcium-fortified tofu, calcium-fortified juices, calcium-fortified rice, soy, and potato drinks

Chloride	Part of hydrochloric acid found in the stomach, necessary for proper digestion	Salt and soy sauce; moderate quantities found in whole, unprocessed foods; large amounts in processed foods
Chromium	Cofactor for insulin	Molasses, nuts, whole grains, and seafood
Copper	Cofactor for enzymes; necessary for iron metabolism; cross-linking of elastin	Liver, shellfish, whole grain cereals, legumes, and nuts
Fluoride	Structural component of calcium hydroxyapatite of bones and teeth	Seafood, meat, fluoridated water
Iodide	A component of the thyroid hormone, thyroxin, which helps to regulate growth, development, and metabolic rate	Iodized salt and seafood
Iron	Structural component of hemoglobin (which carries oxygen in the blood) and myoglobin (which makes oxygen available for muscle contraction) and other enzymes; necessary for the utilization of energy	Red meats, poultry, shellfish, legumes, dried fruits
Magnesium	One of the factors involved in bone mineralization; maintains electrical potential in nerves and muscle membranes; involved in	Widely distributed in most foods; best sources are nuts, fruits, vegetables, and cereals

building of proteins, enzyme action, normal muscular contraction, transmission of nerve impulses, and maintenance of teeth

Manganese	Cofactor for enzymes	Whole grains, green leafy vegetables, and wheat germ
Phosphorus	Bone and teeth formation; regulation of acid-base balance	Milk, poultry, fish, and carbonated beverages
Potassium	Regulation of osmotic pressure and acid-base balance; activation of a number of intracellular enzymes; nerve and muscle contraction	Meats, milk, fruits, vegetables, grains, and legumes
Selenium	Part of glurathione peroxidase (an enzyme that breaks down reactive chemicals that harm cells); works with vitamin E	Seafood, organ meats, muscle meats, grains, and vegetables, depending on soil conditions
Sodium	Regulation of pH, osmotic pressure, and water balance; conductivity or excitability of nerves and muscles; active transport of glucose and amino acids	Salt, soy sauce, seafood, dairy products, and processed foods
Zinc	Part of the hormone insulin and many enzymes; taste perception; wound healing; metabolism of nucleic acids	Red meat, seafood (especially oysters), and beans

Should You Visit a Dietician?

If your child has multiple food allergies or allergies to important foods such as milk and wheat, your physician may suggest a visit to a registered dietician. There are a lot of people out there these days who claim to be dieticians, but only registered dieticians hold bachelor's degrees from an accredited institution, have completed an internship program, passed a comprehensive national exam, and maintain their current registration through continuing education. Your physician probably has a few people to recommend, or you can look for a registered dietician at the American Dietetic Association Web site at www.eatright.org. If you receive a recommendation from a friend or family member, be certain that the dietician has the initials *R.D.* after his or her name and is forthcoming about credentials.

Some parents put off seeing a dietician until their child's height or weight begins to fall, but I think it's certainly easier and better to have that meeting *before* the child's health seems to be compromised. Even if height and weight are not an issue, the nutritional guidance can often be quite valuable. I believe that just picking up two or three really good tips on how to raise the bar nutritionally is worth the generally affordable fee.

Before you have your first appointment with a dietician, you'll need to keep a detailed food diary of everything your child ate or drank over the preceding three to seven days. Because children are small, every mouthful counts. Those five sips of soda and three potato chips cadged from you at lunch may seem insignificant, but over time even little nibbles like that add up. On the plus side, so do the four grapes, the third of a raw carrot, and two bites of meat loaf you may not have considered worthy of notice. Feed your child what you always do and write down everything he or she eats, "good" and "bad," as honestly and accurately as you can. It's not the dietician's role to judge—only to help. (And believe me, they've seen it all, from kids who survive on peanut butter and pretzels to kids who eat only one food for weeks or months at a time.) You may be surprised at how much latitude there is in a healthy diet for children. Pound for pound, growing children need more calories than adults do, and there is room not only for fat (which everyone needs) but for judicious use of treats as well. Using the food diary you've provided, a registered dietician will analyze your child's intake in terms of carbohydrates, protein, fat, vitamins, minerals, and overall caloric value, and make recommendations as necessary.

The dietician's goal is to steer your child's diet toward a healthy, appetizing balance of carbohydrates, proteins (from either animal or plant sources), and fats, which will supply a full range of vitamins and minerals and enough calories to support growth. If there are important foods your child can't or absolutely won't eat, a dietician can recommend the right supplements.

Complex carbohydrates—grains, pasta, potatoes, fruits, and vegetables—are the foundation of a healthy diet, and for most of us, getting enough of them is simple and delicious. But a child who is allergic to wheat and resists your best efforts to serve up the fruits and vegetables may have a harder time of it.

Sugar is a simple carbohydrate. While it doesn't do much for anyone nutritionally, it does supply calories and happiness. When my older son, an indifferent eater as a toddler, would go through a particularly distressing spell of self-imposed starvation, I often found that giving him one small cookie *before* his meal got the juices going enough so that he was willing and able to tackle the lamb chop, baked potato, and broccoli on his tray. Certainly, it doesn't matter when you give the sweet if you've planned on giving it anyway, and it renders the "eat your dinner or you don't get dessert" battle moot from the outset.

Adequate protein is crucial to form muscles, support the rapid growth of a young child's brain, and keep the internal organs functioning. Like carbohydrates, protein comes in many forms. Animal protein—milk, eggs, poultry, fish, seafood, and meat—is convenient because the protein is so high-quality that all of it can be used efficiently by the body. But plant sources of protein—nuts, seeds, legumes, grains, vegetables, and, to a small extent, fruits—can supply the same nutrition with a little extra planning.

Plant proteins are incomplete; they do not supply the full complement of amino acids needed by the body. But combining two or more complementary plant proteins, such as rice and beans or peanut butter on whole wheat bread, yields the same quality protein as an egg, slice of beef, or piece of cheese. If your child, like many, dislikes the taste of meat and cannot eat eggs, milk, or fish, you may find relief from the monotony of chicken, chicken, and more chicken in tasty vegetarian soups, casseroles, side dishes, and spreads. A registered dietician will have immediate suggestions for you, and the abundance of wonderful vegetarian cookbooks available today can supply the rest.

Despite the bad press they've gotten from all corners, not only are fats an important part of a healthy diet, they are essential for optimal brain development in children under the age of two. In fact, experts agree that children under age two should drink whole milk, eat regular ice cream, and enjoy butter, meats, and other high-cholesterol foods without restriction within reasonable limits. Fats make foods taste good, and because they are not as quickly digested as carbohydrates, contribute to a pleasant feeling of prolonged satiety. A child who has had a bit of fat in his or her lunch—mayonnaise in a tuna sandwich, let's say, or a chicken leg with the skin on—will probably not be looking around for an afternoon snack as quickly as the child who ate fat-free turkey breast, whole wheat crackers, and raw vegetables for lunch. (A healthy meal, to be sure, but not one with a lot of staying power.)

Fats are also necessary for proper cell function. Certain vitamins—vitamin E in particular—cannot be absorbed and used by the body in the absence of dietary fat. People who don't get enough fat in their diets (a fairly rare happenstance here in the United States) will often notice that their skin is unpleasantly dry, their digestion is off-kilter, and their energy levels are lower than what they should be.

Of course, this is not an endorsement of rampant, unrestricted fat intake. Obesity is more of a problem for today's children than over-leanness. And not all fats are created equal. Fat comes in three forms: saturated, monosaturated, and polyunsaturated. The saturated fats come primarily from animal sources and are solid at room temperature. Monosaturated and polyunsaturated fats come from plant sources. It is generally agreed that the polyunsaturated fats—those found in oils such as olive oil and canola oil—are the healthiest.

A FINAL WORD OF CAUTION:
MEDICATIONS MAY CONTAIN FOOD TOO

As if monitoring every bite of food weren't hard enough, you also need to know the exact components of every bit of medicine and supplements your child takes when a serious food allergy is present. Wheat in particular may be used as a filler in children's over-the-counter vitamin tablets and other supplements. Milk will sometimes appear in the "inactive ingredients" as lactose or even as sugar. This can be a problem for lactose-intolerant children, whose difficulties are caused by an inability to digest milk sugar, but not for children with true milk allergy. The lactose used in prescription medications is pharmaceutical grade, meaning it is highly standardized and does not contain the milk protein that would cause an allergic reaction. If your child has a severe wheat allergy, it would be a good idea to buy a copy of the *Physician's Desk Reference* and the *Physician's Desk Reference for Non-Prescription Drugs*. Both give detailed information on every drug and are revised each year. To order, call (515) 284-6782.

2

ANAPHYLAXIS

Most parents of allergic children have heard about anaphylaxis. They know it's dangerous, but they don't really know what it is. So they sometimes worry that their child will experience anaphylaxis, but they won't recognize it—and won't treat it in time.

Those of us whose children *have* experienced anaphylaxis have a different take on it entirely: you know it when it happens.

Anaphylaxis literally means "against or without protection." Most doctors reserve the term for a reaction that affects two body systems—hives plus wheezing or vomiting plus wheezing, for example—or any reaction that could escalate into a life-threatening situation. So while a bad bout of eczema or lots of itchy, swollen hives on the trunk are certainly no walk in the park, those symptoms alone do not constitute anaphylaxis. A swelling of the lips and tongue, however, which could impede breathing if allowed to progress, can be considered anaphylaxis.

A child experiencing anaphylaxis may show symptoms in the mouth (a tingling feeling in the mouth is often the first indicator that an allergen is on board), eyes, throat, lungs, stomach, and skin.

Some common symptoms of the anaphylaxis include:

- Itching and swelling of the lips, tongue, inside the mouth, and pharynx (vocal cords). Children may report an itching, burning, or tingling sensation. When symptoms have progressed to include swelling inside the throat, the child's voice begins to grow hoarse, and breathing is accompanied by an audible rasp.
- Widespread hives (urticaria) and skin swelling
- Nausea, vomiting, abdominal pain, and/or diarrhea
- An overall feeling of itchiness, in association with a rash, sneezing, and itchy, runny nose
- Wheezing or a feeling of tightness in the chest
- An anxious, nervous feeling most adults describe as a "sense of impending doom"
- Weakness, fainting, or chest pain, accompanied by a rapid, weak, or irregular pulse
- Shock and loss of consciousness

Gastrointestinal Anaphylaxis

Some parents may notice that a child experiences nausea, vomiting, and/or diarrhea within a few minutes or hours of eating a particular food. While the child is definitely uncomfortable, the symptoms seem to be more of a nuisance than a threat to life. The parents try to avoid the food whenever possible but don't feel particularly alarmed.

Unfortunately, when these symptoms are present, the diagnosis may be gastrointestinal anaphylaxis, which over time can seriously harm a child's health. If the child continues to eat the offending food, the mast cells in the gut become partially desensitized, so he or she may not have as severe a reaction each time. But damage is occurring nonetheless.

Children who have experienced repeated episodes of gastrointestinal anaphylaxis may also come to suffer from malabsorption, intermittent abdominal pain, poor appetite, and weight loss or failure to thrive.

If your child experiences these symptoms after eating a certain food, take them seriously—and make an appointment to discuss them with your pediatrician or allergist.

Depending on the food and your child's immune system, anaphylaxis can be triggered by simply inhaling the cooking fumes of the offending substance or by merely touching the allergenic food and then putting that hand in the mouth. But far more common is the scenario where a child takes one or two nibbles of food and begins to look and feel unwell immediately.

In fact, one of the hallmarks of anaphylaxis is that it usually begins quite quickly; almost always within two hours of eating the offending food. The later the onset of symptoms, the less severe the reaction tends to be.

Like most allergic reactions, anaphylaxis does not usually occur the very first time your child is exposed to a particular food. The problem is, you may not be aware of the prior exposures. If your child has eaten any processed or restaurant food at all, chances are good that he or she has consumed a wide variety of potential allergens, from wheat in soy sauce to ground peanuts or peanut traces in virtually anything. So many allergens—peanut, tree nuts, and soy in particular—"hide" in places where we'd least expect to find them. (See chapter 12, "Hidden Allergens.") Your child may have indeed experienced a mild allergic reaction after eating a certain food for the first time, but a few hives or an episode of vomiting and diarrhea don't immediately send up a red flag for most of us, unless we're already on the lookout for allergic symptoms.

What's more, if you breast-fed your child, he or she was exposed to everything you ate. And there's new evidence to support the theory that fetuses can be sensitized in utero to allergenic foods. In fact, a number of obstetricians and pediatricians have begun recommending that their pregnant patients refrain from eating peanuts or nuts while pregnant and nursing.

PREDISPOSITIONS TO ANAPHYLAXIS

If your child has food allergies but has never had an anaphylactic reaction to one of those foods, you don't have to assume that it's only a matter of time. Not every allergic child—or even most allergic children—will experience anaphylaxis. The following three factors seem to predispose children toward having an anaphylactic reaction.

1. History of eczema or urticaria (hives) as an infant, or a family member who suffers from these conditions. Children who experience anaphylaxis are also more likely to have asthma.

2. Young age. The first two years of life seem to be the "danger zone" for anaphylaxis, particularly for babies who have had widespread eczema. Food allergies in general seem to decrease with age, except for peanut, tree nut, fish, and shellfish allergies.

3. Exposure to different foods. Interestingly enough, the more a population is exposed to a certain food, the greater the chance of individuals developing an allergy to that food. In Scandinavia, where fish is a staple of the diet, an allergy to codfish is fairly common. (Italy and Spain also have relatively high incidences of fish and shellfish allergy.) In China, rice allergy is far more common than it is here in the United States.

In the past two or three generations, peanuts have become a staple food in this country—a jar of peanut butter has pride of place in virtually every pantry. In fact, *as a nation we consume 4 million pounds of peanuts every single day.* So it's no small wonder that the incidence of serious allergic reactions to peanuts has also been on the rise.

The question is, why do peanuts, tree nuts, shellfish, and fish commonly produce such strong, often life-threatening reactions, while other foods we eat every day—bananas, apples, oranges, beef, chicken, potatoes—do not? Theoretically, any and all foods are capable of causing an anaphylactic reaction. There *are* people who cannot eat bananas, for instance, under any circumstances. There just aren't many of them.

The bottom line is, not all allergens are created equal. Some are just more potent than others, capable of causing a reaction with the slightest amount of contact. The foods most likely to cause eczema, hives, swelling, or asthma are the same foods most likely to cause anaphylaxis. They are peanuts, tree nuts, eggs, fish, shellfish, and milk.

TREATING ANAPHYLAXIS

In the United States today, food allergies account for the majority of cases of anaphylaxis seen in hospital emergency rooms. A survey conducted by the Mayo Clinic in 1994 showed that 33 percent of the anaphylactic reactions seen were caused by food—2,740 that year. Of those cases, 135 of the patients died, usually because they were treated with epinephrine too late.

The first line of defense against anaphylaxis is epinephrine. Period. In fact, virtually all deaths associated with anaphylaxis occur because epinephrine is not administered in time. A shot of epinephrine, followed by a dose of liquid antihistamine, is the best combination we have to halt the rapid acceleration of symptoms many children experience when they have an anaphylactic reaction.

Epinephrine is available by prescription only. It comes in two strengths: a "junior" version for children 45 pounds and under (0.15

Facts about Anaphylaxis

1. Although not all anaphylaxis is life threatening, there is no way of predicting what course the anaphylaxis will take. Treat each episode with extreme care.

2. The severity of each anaphylactic episode may vary greatly for many reasons, including the amount of food ingested, how the food was prepared, and if the child is becoming more or less allergic to a particular food.

3. Virtually all anaphylaxis begins within two hours of eating the trigger food, and most episodes begin in less than twenty minutes.

4. In about one of every four episodes of anaphylaxis, the child will have secondary symptoms within three to four hours. It is vital to stay at the E.R. for that length of time.

5. Waiting to treat an anaphylactic reaction and being caught without medication are the biggest factors leading to deaths from anaphylaxis.

6. Most anaphylaxis occurs from "hidden" allergens. Accidents can and do happen at any time.

7. Seventy-five percent of all deaths related to food allergy occur at school.

Anaphylaxis Action Plan

1. Act as quickly as possible at the first symptoms of a reaction.

2. Give your child a shot of epinephrine and a dose of liquid antihistamine as prescribed by your doctor.

3. Call 911.

4. Explain to the dispatcher that your child is experiencing an anaphylactic reaction to food. Quickly describe the symptoms. State that you already gave the child epinephrine and antihistamine, but that you may need more epinephrine as a backup.

5. Stay as calm as possible for your child's sake. If your child has a special toy, doll, or stuffed animal, make sure it's available for comfort.

6. If your state does not authorize emergency personnel to administer epinephrine, ride in the ambulance with your child with an extra dose in case one is needed en route.

7. Keep your child in the E.R. for several hours, as second-phase anaphylactic reactions may occur.

---

mg), and an adult version for children over 45 pounds and adults (0.3 mg). Although it may seem odd that a 45-pound child and a 170-pound man need the same amount of epinephrine, the dosage is actually calculated on surface area. Children have a proportionally higher surface area than adults, so the discrepancy is not as broad as it seems. The medicine is most commonly delivered by a device known as an EpiPen. Each EpiPen delivers one premeasured dose. EpiPens are not reusable and should be thrown away immediately after use.

Perhaps the first time your child had an anaphylactic reaction to food it was treated in the E.R. In such a case, you must see your child's doctor as soon as possible after the incident to discuss what happened, how to avoid it happening again, and to get a prescription for an EpiPen. Most parents need several: two for school (one for the school nurse, one for the classroom teacher) and two for home use are the minimum we would recommend for a school-age child. You definitely need access to two EpiPens at any given time, however. Think of the possible scenarios: one EpiPen might malfunction (this is quite rare, but it does happen occasionally, whether because of a manufacturing defect or because of exposure to temperature extremes), or one EpiPen might not be enough to reverse your child's reaction. Epinephrine generally lasts for twenty minutes or less, so you might need to give your child a second injection before you reach the E.R.

If your child has ever experienced an anaphylactic reaction to food, both epinephrine and liquid antihistamine (with a medicine measuring cup) should always be close at hand and brought with you wherever you go, even if you're sure your child won't be eating. This isn't being paranoid; it's being practical. Allergic substances such as peanuts can turn up virtually anywhere: a bit of crumbled peanut on a movie theater seat; crumbs from a peanut butter cookie in a grocery cart seat; a tiny dab of peanut butter on the hand of your child's new playground friend, peanut shells that your child may pick up at the playground. Other substances such as milk, wheat, tree nuts, and egg may be encountered in much the same ways.

Assume the worst, and pack accordingly. Put your medications in a special bag and keep them in your handbag or someplace where you have immediate access to them at all times. A friend of mine keeps an extra EpiPen and bottle of Benadryl prominently displayed in a see-through plastic bag on a hook in her garage, so her husband will always see the bag and grab it before taking their son anywhere in the car. Another friend keeps hers on the kitchen counter at all times. I simply keep mine in my handbag and make sure that my handbag is always close to *me*.

THE PROGRESS OF ANAPHYLAXIS

When your child—let's say it's your son—eats a food he is severely allergic to, the immune system responds by pouring out a combination of chemicals, including those famous bad guys, histamines. Within minutes, or even seconds, the first symptoms of anaphylaxis appear. (They may be as innocent as a major bout of sneezing or as serious as difficulty breathing.)

Your son's lips and tongue may swell, resulting in a form of "deep-seated" hives known as angiodema. His face and throat may swell, signaling an enlargement and "leaking" of the blood vessels in this area. He may complain of an itchy feeling in the throat or may feel the throat start to close up. He may break out in large, intensely itchy hives all over the body, which after a certain amount of time blend together, looking like a badly swollen sunburn. You may notice that your son's nose is running, and that he is starting to wheeze and show symptoms of excessive phlegm production and tissue swelling. He may vomit.

One thing you can count on: anaphylaxis progresses rapidly. Therefore immediate treatment is the name of the game.

Exercise-induced Anaphylaxis

Some people feel fine when they eat a certain food and fine when they exercise, but if they eat that particular food *and* exercise immediately after, they experience a syndrome known as exercise-induced anaphylaxis. Needless to say, this type of anaphylaxis can be baffling to the people involved and baffling to diagnose: in most cases, the food implicated had been eaten by the patient for much of his or her life with no ill effect. It was only when exercise was added to the equation that the reaction occurred. Luckily, exercise-induced anaphylaxis is not common. But as with all other serious allergic reactions, people who have experienced exercise-induced anaphylaxis need to be careful about what they eat and have epinephrine available at all times.

If your son does not receive treatment, and the anaphylaxis continues to progress (not all anaphylaxis progresses relentlessly toward disaster, but you have no way of knowing if it will or won't), blood will pool in the arms and legs, depriving the heart and brain of oxygen. At this point, your son will be slipping into shock. Loss of consciousness and death may follow.

Like all allergic reactions, the symptoms of anaphylaxis differ from child to child. But once a child has had a particular reaction, he or she will often react in a similar way. Children who have experienced closing of the throat in reaction to eggs, for example, are likely to have that reaction when they ingest egg protein again. The only difference may lie in how quickly the reaction begins and how severe it is. If, for example, your daughter accidentally eats a whole egg (disguised as French toast), the reaction will be much worse than if she ate a packaged cookie that contained trace amounts of egg yolk.

HOW EPINEPHRINE AND ANTIHISTAMINE WORK

When you give your child a shot of epinephrine (also sold under the brand names AnaKit and AnaGuard), the immediate effect is an overall constricting of the blood vessels and a stronger, faster heartbeat. The bronchial tubes enlarge as well.

Once those blood vessels go back to normal size, the swelling that is the most alarming (and life-threatening) symptom of anaphylaxis rapidly abates. Swollen airways open up; lips and tongue shrink back

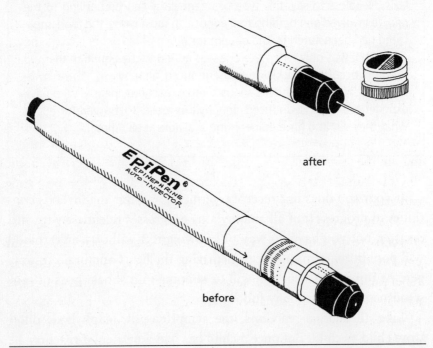

after

before

Before it has been used (larger drawing), an EpiPen is pretty much the same size and shape as a large Magic Marker. After it has been injected and withdrawn, you can see the fine needle.

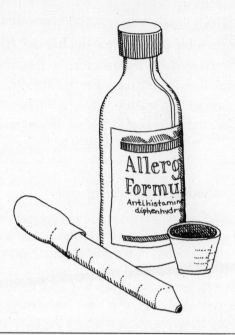

When you're dealing with an allergic reaction, liquid antihistamine (as opposed to tablets) works fastest. Be sure to always have a measuring cup or dropper on hand to deliver the correct dose.

to normal; wheezing is replaced by easy breathing. The risk of shock has been averted; with blood vessels back to normal, blood goes where it's supposed to go—to the heart and brain—rather than pooling in the extremities. In fact, anyone who has experienced the "before" and "after" of a reaction that was treated with epinephrine can attest to its near-miraculous properties.

The importance of epinephrine as the line of first defense in anaphylaxis really can't be overstated. Nothing can replace it. If your child is wheezing, asthma medicines may provide some measure of relief (or, depending on how severe the reaction is, they may not offer any at all), but they have no effect whatsoever on the swelling of blood vessels elsewhere in the body. Without epinephrine, your child could still go into shock.

The moral of the story is, give your child epinephrine at the first signs of a serious allergic reaction. The pattern of every child's reaction is unique. If your child has experienced anaphylaxis before, you know what symptoms to expect. Use common sense, as well. If your nut-allergic child takes a big bite of a granola bar and starts to swell up, assume that the granola bar was somehow contaminated with nuts even if none were listed in the ingredients. Give the epinephrine. It won't cause any damage if it wasn't truly needed, but you may not be able to stop a devastating reaction in time if you wait too long.

About EpiPen Auto-Injector

If the thought of using an EpiPen makes you queasy, just think about the alternative: a long-needled syringe. The EpiPen Auto-Injector as we know it was originally developed by the military during World War I as an antidote to nerve gas, although it was not available to the public until some years later. Its convenient format and quick delivery of medicine were a godsend for soldiers who were already under intense stress. And while we parents are not under quite the same acute pressure, no one can deny that we're fighting our own battle in the trenches.

Unfortunately, epinephrine is not a stable drug. If it gets too hot or too cold, it will not be effective. Here are some guidelines to keep your epinephrine fresh and ready to use.

• Make sure that epinephrine is stored as close to room temperature as possible at all times. Refrigeration or exposure to prolonged cold may cause the unit to malfunction. When traveling outside with epinephrine during the winter—while skiing, for example—you should keep the EpiPen in a breast pocket or in a waist pocket under your jacket.

• Your EpiPen should also not be exposed to extreme heat. During the summer, it's important not to store your EpiPen in the glove compartment or trunk of your car. (Of course, it should be with you at all times, anyway.) At the beach, keep your epinephrine in a cooler. Walking around on a hot summer day with epinephrine in your handbag is OK.

• Do not expose your EpiPen to direct sunlight. It will oxidize (turn dark) and not be effective.

• Epinephrine is perishable; check the expiration date every few months to make sure that you don't get caught short.

• Also check your EpiPen every few months to make sure it hasn't oxidized for whatever reason. If the liquid has turned dark, you need to get a new EpiPen.

Dr. Hugh Sampson reports that he has seen far too many children show up at the E.R. in very bad shape, simply because their parents were afraid to give the EpiPen injection. They had the epinephrine; they just wouldn't use it. All of us can empathize with what those moms were going through, but as the saying goes, "You gotta do what you gotta do." The injection itself does not hurt that much—it's the idea of a "shot" that frightens most children (and their parents, for that matter).

An EpiPen could very well save your child's life, but unfortunately, like too much coffee, epinephrine may make a youngster jittery, jumpy, and a bit hyperactive for a while. Some kids seem extremely anxious and uncomfortable; others less so. This period of intense discomfort doesn't generally last more than fifteen minutes, but this can feel like a very long time. Don't be surprised if your child vomits. The important thing to remember is that the injection is an essential step toward recovery.

How to Give an EpiPen Injection

1. Although the EpiPen Auto-Injector may be used through clothing, it's preferable to use it on bare skin. If you are out in public when a reaction occurs, quickly usher your child out of the thick of things and remove his or her pants or leggings as discreetly as possible.

2. Remove the EpiPen from its packaging.

3. Pull off the gray safety cap.

4. Place the black tip on the outer thigh or front of the thigh. *Never inject into a vein or into buttocks!*

5. Push EpiPen Auto-Injector against thigh until unit activates, and hold in place while counting to ten. The full dose of medicine will be fully discharged within a few seconds. If you have practiced with EpiPen trainers in the past, understand that you will not hear a "click" when you are using a real EpiPen.

6. When you remove the EpiPen, you will see the needle protruding. Cap the EpiPen and discard.

7. Don't be concerned if you see some medicine left in the EpiPen. That is normal.

Calling 911

When your child is experiencing an anaphylactic reaction, it is imperative to let the emergency technicians know what they'll be dealing with. This sample phone script gives all the necessary information in a few clear sentences:

"Hello, my name is _____, at (address). My _____-year-old child is experiencing an anaphylactic allergic reaction to (food). I have already given him/her a shot of epinephrine and some liquid antihistamine. Please send your people as quickly as possible, and *tell them to bring more epinephrine with them.* My child requires a _____ dose of epinephrine. (Generally, children who weigh forty-five pounds and under require the junior dose, and those over forty-five pounds need the adult dose.)

Once your child can comfortably swallow, it's important to follow up with a liquid antihistamine such as Benadryl. Liquid antihistamines, as opposed to tablets, are the drug of choice because they begin to work almost immediately. But if you're in a pinch, opt for the tablets rather than offering no antihistamine at all.

Antihistamines work by "fooling" the histamine receptors in your child's body. They have been manufactured to be so like the allergy symptom–producing histamines that the histamine receptors pick them up. But because they are not histamines, they do not cause a reaction. In effect, they block a reaction. So clearly, the sooner your child receives antihistamine, the better, because fewer histamines will have reached their targets and produced troubling symptoms such as hives, excess phlegm, and overall itchiness. Once the antihistamine has taken effect, the histamine symptoms will recede. As with epinephrine, the improvement can seem miraculous. (I plan on writing a note of appreciation to the makers of Benadryl, which has helped my son through many an uncomfortable reaction.)

Don't Leave Home without It!

If your child has ever experienced an anaphylactic reaction, even if it was only once, you should never leave home without:

1. EpiPen and Benadryl. Make sure your EpiPen is the right dosage and has not expired. Pack a teaspoon or measuring cup for the Benadryl.

2. An action plan. (See page 54.) It can be hard to think clearly when you're in a crisis situation. Include a copy of your action plan in your medication bag, and you won't have to remember phone numbers or worry about forgetting something.

3. A MedicAlert bracelet or necklace for your child. Medical personnel are trained to look for these identifying tags when treating any admission. And if the unthinkable happens—your child becomes lost, or you become incapacitated and cannot speak for your child—the MedicAlert emblem will say what you cannot.

WHEN SHOULD YOU GO TO THE E.R.?

The first time your child has an allergic reaction that's more severe than eczema, mild hives, minor gastrointestinal symptoms, or some nasal congestion, you should probably go to the E.R. Any threat to respiration—prolonged coughing or any wheezing or throat tightness—warrants a prompt visit, as does any swelling of the lips and tongue. Allergic reactions can progress in unpredictable ways, and there's no good reason to stay put just waiting to see how ill your child may become. He or she may become very ill in a relatively short amount of time, in which case you need to be where treatment is readily available. Then again, the symptoms may resolve on their own and your child may be just fine—in which case you merely erred on the side of caution, a perfectly justifiable parental instinct.

If you're on the fence, quickly throw together a few books or other amusements for your child and consider going to the E.R. waiting room. If a reaction does indeed seem to be gaining momentum, you're right where you should be. If after waiting a reasonable amount of time no reaction occurs, you can always go home. Don't think of the hour or two you spent there as wasted, but rather as *invested* in your child's safety.

Don't let fear of embarrassment or the sense that you ought to be able to "tough it out" stand in the way of bringing your child to the E.R. if you feel that the trip is in the least bit warranted. People show up there all the time with far milder complaints than your child's.

I now know from personal experience that if Lucas were ever to experience an anaphylactic reaction when I was alone with him, I would call 911 rather than attempt to drive him to the E.R. myself. For one thing, I would hate the thought of him alone in the back of the car without somebody beside him to hold his hand; for another, I would probably be too shaky to drive. (Remember Driver's Ed, when the instructor taught you not to drive if you were under severe emotional duress?) I would also think about the red lights and traffic jams I might encounter along the way, which an ambulance can power right through.

There is a tendency among many of us to think of the E.R. as the place of last resort, to be visited only in cases of serious injury or heart attacks. But here is a simple rule of thumb to follow: any time you need to administer epinephrine, you also need to make a trip to the E.R. Epinephrine is a short-acting medication, frequently offering only fifteen minutes of coverage. Backup doses may be needed. There is also the possibility that your child will experience a second-phase reaction that should be treated and monitored in a hospital setting. Children should be observed for at least four hours, and occasionally as long as six hours, to make sure they don't experience a second stage of the reaction or a delayed reaction. Do everyone a favor, and stay in the E.R. for the length of time that the staff deems necessary. They've dealt with this situation before.

Once you're at the E.R., if your child's reaction does continue to progress, or if he or she has a second-phase reaction, doctors will be on hand with the appropriate medications. Sometimes a child requires a second shot of epinephrine. A child with asthma may need bronchodialators or oxygen. Hives can reappear for days following an allergic reaction, and will need to be treated with additional doses of antihistamine.

Of course, if you know that your child should have epinephrine and for whatever reason it is not on hand when a reaction begins, *you must go to the E.R. at once.*

If your child has asthma, and begins to experience wheezing in conjunction with any other allergic symptoms, administer epinephrine and get to the E.R. right away. Children with asthma have what's known as a reactive airway. Unfortunately, it seldom reacts in ways that lead to health and well-being. Although the number of people in the United States who die from food allergies each year is not considered that high—about 125 in all—people with asthma account for most of the victims.

AVOIDING ANAPHYLAXIS

If you're wondering why you never heard about such serious food reactions when *you* were a kid, you're not alone. The first time a description of food-induced anaphylaxis appeared in the medical literature was 1969. Researchers debate why the incidence of food-induced anaphylaxis appears to be on the rise, but there's no debating the fact that it is. Most of the increase is in peanut-related reactions, and the growing infiltration of peanuts into our food supply could certainly be the chief reason.

Children who have experienced anaphylaxis once have already ably demonstrated their ability to do so. (Not all children, not even children with multiple food allergies, will anaphylax. It's an innate talent, like perfect pitch or a photographic memory.) Naturally, having lived through one such harrowing episode, both children and their parents are loath to repeat it.

Complete and total avoidance of the offending food will keep your child safe from that particular reaction. If your child is very young—infant through preschool—and has not yet been exposed to foods such as peanuts, shellfish, or tree nuts, it may not be a bad idea to hold off on introducing them at this stage of the game.

Researchers agree that once a child has had an anaphylactic reaction to a particular food—severe hives and wheezing in reaction to peanuts, for example—he or she will often repeat that pattern upon subsequent exposures. The only difference in the reaction may lie in its severity, depending upon how much of the allergen was actually ingested. For example, a severely peanut-allergic girl who takes one tiny bite of a peanut butter cookie by mistake will generally *not* get as sick as she would have had the whole cookie been eaten. However, even the tiny bite will probably cause a reaction that requires medication right away.

I've said it before, but I'll say it again: *If your child has had an anaphylactic reaction to any food, he or she must completely and totally avoid that food at all times.*

Finally, under the category of "Mixed Blessing," I submit this anecdote:

Lucas was taking a group swimming lesson at our local Y, and he loved everything about it. So I felt comfortable sitting and chatting with the other moms at the far end of the pool. I'd glance over every five minutes or so to see what he was doing, but my attention was definitely more focused on my friends.

All of a sudden my friend Amy (who, bless her heart, kept a sharper eye on the water) turned white. "Oh my God," she said, covering her mouth and pointing. There was Lucas being led by his teacher toward me. Blood poured down his face. His face and chest were covered with it.

I made it to my feet and trotted over to meet them halfway, towel in hand. Kneeling by Lucas, I started clearing the blood, gently probing for the wound. "What happened?" I asked the shaken teacher. "I don't know" was the reply. "He was doing bobs and must have hit his head on the side of the pool."

Aha! There it was, up by his hairline: a jagged, ugly gash about an inch wide and almost an inch deep. "You're going to need some stitches, honey," I told Lucas. "We need to take you to the doctor right away."

"OK, Mommy," Lucas agreed, blood still streaking down his face. "I'll get stitches. *After* I finish my swimming lesson."

I had to laugh. Just then, my friend Amy approached us. "Is he OK?" she asked, fear tightening her voice.

"He's fine," I said, realizing with amazement that I really did believe it. "He's *breathing*. He's *conscious*. I don't need to give him epinephrine and call 911 and pray that the ambulance gets here right away. We're cool."

Lucas ended up needing twenty-four stitches, three layers of eight stitches each, but I was able to stay calm—and most important, keep *him* feeling as calm as possible.

I'd had a look at death once. This wasn't it.

Once you've dealt with anaphylaxis, almost anything else feels like small stuff.

ACTION PLAN FOR DAY CARE, SCHOOL, OR CAMP

The form on page 54 is the standard version developed by the Food Allergy Network. It has space for all the information necessary to correctly treat a child during an allergic emergency.

THE MEDICALERT FOUNDATION

Although there are a number of organizations that can provide identifying emblems and some support services, MedicAlert is generally recognized as offering the most comprehensive coverage in an emergency situation. Founded by a physician whose daughter almost died from an allergic reaction, the MedicAlert Foundation now has nearly 2.3 million members nationwide.

The MedicAlert emblem, engraved with your child's personal ID number and essential medical information, may be worn as a bracelet or as a necklace. When an emergency worker sees the emblem, he or she knows to immediately call MedicAlert's twenty-four-hour Emergency Response Center to receive all the vital information about your child's allergy and any other ongoing medical problems.

EMERGENCY HEALTH CARE PLAN

Place Child's Picture Here

Allergy To: _____

Student's

Name: _____ D.O.B.: ___ Teacher: _____

Asthmatic   Yes ❑*   No ❑
        *High risk for severe reaction

SIGNS OF AN ALLERGIC REACTION INCLUDE:

Systems   *Symptom*

• MOUTH   itching and swelling of the lips, tongue, or mouth

• THROAT[†]   itching and/or a sense of tightness in the throat, hoarseness, and
             hacking cough

• SKIN   hives, itchy rash, and/or swelling about the face or extremities

• GUT   nausea, abdominal cramps, vomiting, and/or diarrhea

• LUNG[†]   shortness of breath, repetitive coughing, and/or wheezing

• HEART[†]   "thready" pulse, "passing-out"

The severity of symptoms can change quickly.
[†]All above symptoms can potentially progress to a life-threatening situation!

ACTION:

1. If ingestion is suspected, give _____
                                      medication/dose/route

   and _____ immediately!

2. CALL RESCUE SQUAD: _____.

3. CALL: Mother _____ Father _____ or emergency contacts.

4. CALL: Dr. _____ at _____.

**DO NOT HESITATE TO ADMINISTER MEDICATION OR CALL RESCUE SQUAD
EVEN IF PARENTS OR DOCTOR CANNOT BE REACHED!**

_____ _____ _____ M.D. _____
Parent's Signature   Date   Doctor's Signature   Date

Emergency Contacts	Trained Staff Members
1. _____	1. _____ Room _____
Relation: _____ Phone: _____	
2. _____	2. _____ Room _____
Relation: _____ Phone: _____	
3. _____	3. _____ Room _____
Relation: _____ Phone: _____	

For children with multiple food allergies, use one form for each food.

3

MILK

We produce over 60 million tons of milk each year in the United States, with three-quarters of that consumed as fluid milk or cheese. There's no denying that we're a nation of dairy lovers. We'll have a bowl of cereal with milk in the morning, a cheeseburger and chocolate shake at noon, milk and cookies after school, and steak and baked potatoes (with sour cream or butter, of course) followed by a dish of ice cream at night.

But milk is such a common source of allergies or discomfort for young children—it's estimated that 2.5 percent of babies and toddlers are affected—that it's often the first food pediatricians recommend eliminating when a child has chronic eczema, hives, wheezing not caused by illness, a runny nose, or a tummy problem.

A specific kind of allergic reaction that's confined to the gastrointestinal tract is called enterocolitis. If your child has it, chances are you've known that something was going on since he or she was a newborn. Babies with enterocolitis experience vomiting, diarrhea, or both when they ingest milk protein.

For most milk allergies, doctors suggest trying a soy-based formula, and if that proves undoable or unsatisfactory, they'll recom-

Milk Alert!

The following terms on an ingredients label indicate the presence of milk. Avoid them!

Artificial butter flavor
Butter, butter fat, butter oil
Buttermilk
Casein
Caseinates (listed as ammonium, calcium, magnesium, potassium, or sodium caseinate)
Cheese and cottage cheese
Cream
Curds
Custard
Ghee
Half and half
Hydrolysates (listed as casein, milk protein, protein, whey, or whey protein hydrolysate)
Lactalbumin, lactalbumin phosphate
Lactoglobulin
Lactose
Lactulose
Milk (derivative, powder, protein, solids, malted, condensed, evaporated, dry, whole, low-fat, nonfat, skimmed, and goat's milk)
Nougat
Pudding
Rennet casein
Sour cream, sour cream solids
Sour milk solids
Whey (in all forms, including sweet, delactosed, and protein concentrate)
Yogurt

The following terms *may* indicate the presence of milk:

Chocolate
Flavorings, including caramel, Bavarian cream, coconut cream, brown sugar, butter, and natural flavorings
High protein flour
Margarine
Simplesse

mend a hypoallergenic formula, which consists of milk protein that's been so broken down that it's virtually undetectable by the immune system. About 15 percent of children who are allergic to cow's milk are also allergic to soy formula. (Kids with at least one allergy have already proved that they have an overreactive immune system, after all.) Children with enterocolitis, on the other hand, run such a high risk of being allergic to soy formula—about 50 percent—that the wisest course is to go straight for the hypoallergenic formula.

Switching infants or toddlers to a different formula is usually pretty easy to do (yes, I know it smells bad to you, but after a quick adjustment your baby will think it's just fine), and both the soy and hypoallergenic versions are just as nutritious as standard milk-based formulas. But for older children, who have already discovered the joys of grilled cheese, buttered waffles, ice cream, hot cocoa, and pizza—not to mention the scads of cookies, cakes, candies, snack foods, and other goodies made with milk—eliminating milk can be more of a challenge.

It's important here to make a firm distinction between a true milk allergy, which is an immune system response, and lactose intolerance, which is a digestive problem. A child with a true milk allergy (or one whose pediatrician suspects to have a milk allergy) should completely

---

Physical Signs of Milk Allergy

Some babies and young children who are allergic to milk may not have the distinctive signs of eczema or asthma, but wear the evidence plain as day nonetheless. You may see any or all of these signs:

- Dark blue, black, or reddish circles under the eyes (known as "allergic shiners")
- Reddish earlobes
- A reddened nose (which is the result of constantly rubbing the tip up and down to stop the itch, a movement known as the "allergic salute")

avoid any and all forms of milk and milk protein, from the most obvious (a slice of cheese) to the most subtle (casein, a milk protein, in a product touted as "lactose-free"). For milk-allergic children, complete and total avoidance of all milk products is not only the key to health but offers the best chance of eventually outgrowing the allergy completely.

MILK ALLERGY VERSUS LACTOSE INTOLERANCE

Children with lactose intolerance, on the other hand, don't need to avoid milk products at all—they just need to stick to the lactose-reduced or lactose-free versions, or take a tablet containing the lactase enzyme before eating dairy foods. (These are widely available in pharmacies and grocery stores. Consult your pediatrician as to the proper dosage.) Lactose intolerance varies widely from child to child. Many kids are fine having one glass of milk and a few slices of cheese a day, and run into trouble only when they consume more than that.

Get R.E.A.L. about Medications

Read Every and All Labels applies to everything that goes into your child's mouth, from lollipops to french fries to medicine.

Lactose is frequently added to both prescription and over-the-counter medications to make the products tastier or give them bulk. Currently, manufacturers of pharmaceuticals are not required by law to specifically list milk as an ingredient, although some do. Sometimes when sugar is listed as an active agent, it could be lactose, which is milk sugar. This will not cause a problem for a milk-allergic child but could make a severely lactose-intolerant child ill.

If you have doubts about the safety of a particular medicine, the best recourse is to contact the pharmaceutical company directly and explain your concerns. Chances are you will receive a prompt and courteous reply that will clear up the mystery once and for all.

Beef Alert!

Although it is not common, some children who are highly allergic to milk will develop an allergic reaction to beef as well. The beef reaction can be just as severe as the milk allergy and usually shows up within two hours of eating. In the unusual event that your child experiences symptoms typical of his or her milk allergy after eating a beef meal (and you are absolutely certain that the meal was dairy-free), you can probably assume that beef was the culprit.

If your child has not experienced any problems with beef, there is no need to eliminate it. Most milk-allergic children will not develop a beef allergy. In fact, since many milk-allergic children have an egg allergy as well, beef becomes an even more important source of protein, vitamins, and minerals in the diet.

Other kids start feeling crampy and bloated from a small scoop of ice cream. You probably have a good idea of your child's limit, but if you don't, it's well worth the time to keep a food diary for a few weeks and note how your child reacts to different amounts and types of dairy foods.

There doesn't seem to be any correlation between milk allergy and lactose intolerance. Kids who have milk allergies now are no more likely to develop lactose intolerance later in life than the general population. (But the general population is highly likely to: about 80 percent of us are lacking in the lactase enzyme to various degrees.) Lactose intolerance is most widespread among African Americans, Jews, Asians, and people of Mediterranean descent.

All that being said, milk is a valuable food. Along with its universal appeal (and near-universal appearance in foods dear to children), milk puts hefty doses of protein and calcium in your child's diet, as well as riboflavin, pantothenic acid, phosphorus, and vitamin D. But milk is not the only source of these nutrients. The protein, riboflavin, pantothenic acid, and phosphorus are easy enough to replace if your child eats eggs, meat, chicken, or fish—or enjoys a well-balanced vegetarian diet, with plenty of legumes, nuts, seeds, and whole grains. The vitamin D can come from direct sunlight (fifteen minutes a day or more without sunscreen, not necessarily advisable for fair-skinned children) or from vitamin supplements. And happily, the calcium is easier to replace than ever before.

CALCIUM REPLACEMENTS

Growing bones need calcium and plenty of it every day. In the first year of life, children require 600 mg of calcium daily. Kids between the ages of one and twelve need 800 mg daily. Teenagers should have a whopping 1,200 mg a day. Acknowledging the fact that most Americans don't get enough calcium in their diets—and are increasingly concerned about it—many food manufacturers are adding calcium to their products. Other foods that we don't ordinarily think of as being rich in calcium turn out to have a fair share. Here are just some of the sources:

• Calcium-enriched juices, particularly orange juice, which can offer as much calcium as a glass of milk. Serve a tall glass of calcium-fortified OJ at breakfast, then follow up with calcium-fortified juice boxes (or more OJ) at snack time and lunch. If your child doesn't like orange juice, substitute calcium-fortified apple, grape, and fruit punch versions. Your rule of thumb should be to serve only the juices that have calcium added.

• Calcium-enriched cereals. Many cereals on the shelves now display the banner "A good source of calcium." Upon closer inspection, you'll notice that one serving seldom offers more than 10 percent of the daily quota. A few of the multigrain cereals offer 25 percent. However, since most children eat more than a single serving at a sitting, calcium-fortified cereals are a good deal, especially when served with calcium-fortified beverages. (Be sure the cereals are dairy-free, of course.)

• Nondairy calcium-enriched beverages made from rice or soy. The soy beverages are higher in protein than the rice beverages, but if your child can't have soy or dislikes the taste, the rice beverages are a fine milk substitute.

• Calcium-enriched baked goods. Many health food stores offer calcium-enriched muffins, waffles, and other breakfast treats that are happily free of milk and eggs. They tend to be on the expensive side, but many parents think that they're worth it. If you can find a brand that your child likes, you may be able to meet a full third of his or her calcium quota with a single serving.

• Green leafy vegetables, though not a tremendous source of calcium, contribute their fair share. Kale, in particular, is loaded with calcium.

• Canned salmon with the bones is an easy way to get calcium into many children. Mash the salmon well and mix with bread crumbs and egg (or a little salad dressing if egg is a problem) to make fried salmon croquettes, which most children love. Or make salmon salad sandwiches. Sardines with the bones are a good source of calcium as well.

• Some pediatricians recommend Tums, which are high in calcium, for their milk-allergic or milk-averse patients. Taken with meals, this product can help make up a calcium deficit for many children. Ask your pediatrician or allergist what his/her thoughts are on the matter.

• Stay on the lookout for calcium-fortified products at the supermarket—new ones are coming on the market all the time. Just be sure to carefully read the ingredients, as many do contain dairy.

But right now, the best thing you can do for your child is to restructure his or her diet to completely eliminate any traces of milk protein.

Eliminating milk from your child's diet is equal parts avoidance and substitution. It's not easy, but it won't be terrible, either. Be sure to read chapter 12, "Hidden Allergens," for a complete discussion of how and where milk protein can sneak into your child's diet, and how to steer clear of those situations. The accompanying table will help you get started with milk substitutes. I like to think of it as the Milk-Free Parallel Universe.

INSTEAD OF THIS DAIRY FOOD:	TRY THIS NONDAIRY FOOD:
Milk for drinking or pouring on cereal	Calcium-enriched soy or rice milk, soy formula, or other nondairy formula. For chocolate milk, add one teaspoon of unsweetened cocoa plus sugar to taste.
Cheese	Vegan (no animal products at all) cheese, sold at a few health food stores. Read the label carefully. Soy cheeses and other "nondairy" cheeses contain milk protein and should be avoided.
Ice cream	Soy- or rice-based frozen desserts, sorbets, frozen rice-based puddings, frozen juice pops. Read all labels carefully for every product. And remember, many brands of ice cream cones and sprinkles are dairy-free!
Yogurt	A smoothie. Follow the recipe on page 64 and freeze until partly set.
Butter	Dairy-free margarine for cooking, eating, and baking; dairy-free shortening for baking.
Chocolate	National and store brands of dairy-free semisweet chocolate, most often available as chocolate chips. For a special treat, melt the chocolate, stir in crisp rice cereal, spread in a greased pan to cool, and then cut into pieces.
Liquid milk in baking	The same quantity of the milk substitute of your choice, or apple juice plus one tablespoon of oil.

GETTING READY FOR DAIRY-FREE LIVING

Make a trip to the grocery store, preferably alone, so you'll have plenty of time to carefully read all the labels before making your food selections. Fortunately, you can choose from a variety of national brands. You'll need to buy:

- Milk-free bread
- Milk-free cereal
- Milk-free breadstuffs, such as crackers and pretzels
- Milk-free desserts (including ice pops and sorbets—*not* sherbet— milk-free "ice creams" and "puddings," and gelatin desserts)
- Milk-free chocolate chips and unsweetened cocoa for the fabulous chocolate chip cookies and cake that you can make by following the recipes in chapter 16
- Milk-free margarine
- Milk-free pancake and muffin mixes, if your family enjoys them
- Treat food for older children, such as fruit chews and lollipops (use on an as-needed basis—especially when the neighbor kid appears at your front door eating a chocolate bar)

Breakfast and dessert time are usually the hardest parts of the day for a milk-allergic child. If your child can have rice milk or soy milk, and will accept it in cereal, a good deal of your breakfast problem is solved.

When it comes to making substitutions in baking, I've found that it's a lot easier to work with milk substitutes than with egg substitutes. The leavening action is unaffected, and in many cases the difference is indiscernible. Some recipes come out better with solid shortening such as Crisco (not the butter-flavored kind, and please be sure to read the ingredients on each and every package you buy!) than they do with milk-free margarine. Cookies like ginger snaps, for example, that are supposed to have a crackle top, are usually better with Crisco.

Here are some more suggestions for milk-free eating.

• To thicken soups or give sauces a rich finish, make a roux: Starting with one tablespoon of each, combine milk-free margarine with flour in a small bowl, and cut in until mixture resembles coarse crumbs. If you have time, brown the mixture in a small skillet. If you're in a hurry, add a little of the liquid you're cooking with to the roux, and mix until dissolved. When the mixture is the consistency of smooth applesauce, you've got it right. Stir the roux, a little bit at a time, into your sauce until no lumps remain. As the sauce cooks, it will continue to thicken, so be conservative. Cook the sauce for an additional ten minutes to eliminate any possible "raw flour" taste.

• Make mashed potatoes with olive oil, salt, and pepper and a little crushed garlic. Or make mashed sweet potatoes instead, with cinnamon, sugar, and some fruit preserves. (Apricot is especially tasty.) Children who think mashed potatoes are "icky" often change their tune when the potatoes are reheated in individual ramekins.

• Another nice thickener that lends a creamy taste to soups and stews and packs a vitamin-filled punch is a vegetable puree. Simply peel and chop a potato, two parsnips, two carrots, and an onion. Put in a bowl with one-half cup of water, and microwave on high power for twenty to twenty-five minutes. Pour everything plus at least an additional half cup of water or chicken broth into a blender, and blend until smooth. I use this puree as a soup base to thicken beef, chicken, or vegetable broth. It's also wonderful for pot roast.

• Fruit smoothies are a delicious alternative to milk shakes. Our favorite recipe is one cup of calcium-fortified orange juice, one ripe banana, three or four big, juicy strawberries, and a squirt of honey. Blend until completely smooth and enjoy! To serve as a dessert, just pour the mixture into plastic ice pop holders and freeze until firm. You can also make a smoothie with soy milk, for an added protein boost.

• Frozen bananas have a surprisingly creamy taste. On a stick, they're a real treat—especially if you let your child roll them in honey, raisins, and whatever other allowable goodies your imagination comes up with.

A Cautionary Tale for Parents of Highly Milk-Allergic Children

If you have used powdered milk in the past, you may want to think twice about preparing it while your milk-allergic child is home. We recently heard about a little girl who was watching TV in the family room while her mother prepared powdered milk in the kitchen. Within moments the little girl suffered an anaphylactic reaction. Apparently, enough of the milk powder had become airborne to seriously affect her.

PAREVE FOODS

Observant Jews obey dietary laws known as *kashruth*. They keep kosher, meaning, among other things, that they never mix milk with meat at the same meal. This comes from the biblical injunction to "not boil a kid in its mother's milk." People who are kosher don't use the same pots, dishes, or utensils to prepare and eat dairy products as they do to eat meat; they don't even store them in the same cabinets.

Cheeseburgers, steak with a buttered potato, a glass of milk with a roast beef sandwich—none of these foods are allowed in a kosher home. Even a dish of ice cream for dessert after a meat meal is considered too close for comfort. So naturally, it's vitally important for kosher people to know when purchasing packaged foods if the items contain milk or not.

Many national brands are marked with kosher symbols. A *U* in a circle or the word *pareve* (also spelled *parve*) means that the food is considered to have neither meat nor milk elements in it, and can therefore be consumed as part of either a meat or a dairy meal. (Fruits and vegetables, fish, eggs, grain products, nuts, and many candies fall into this category.)

There was a time when those of us with milk-allergic children considered ourselves to be home free when we saw those friendly little markings. After all, a rabbi was right there at the plant, carefully supervising the whole production process! And for most of us, whose children's milk allergies were not life threatening, the *U* symbol, combined with a thorough reading of the ingredients, was indeed a good guide.

Unfortunately, a food that qualifies as pareve is not necessarily completely and totally free of milk protein. Religion can allow a few milligrams here and there to pass through, but immune systems cannot. Children who are extremely sensitive to milk, or anaphylactic to milk, may have a reaction to one or some of the ingredients. Let's say, for example, that the item in question is a semisweet chocolate bar. Although the machine the chocolate bar is processed on may be devoted solely to this particular kind of candy, some of the cocoa used in making the chocolate may have been processed at a plant that also processes a milk chocolate mixture on the same line. The line may have been carefully cleaned out to the rabbi's satisfaction, but let's face it: short of climbing in there with a Q-tip and scrubbing every single square inch, there's no way to completely and totally eliminate every speck of milk chocolate.

Another kosher marking you may see is *D.E.*, meaning "dairy equipment." The food itself may be dairy-free, but the equipment it is processed on also processes milk-containing foods. Frequently, the only difference between pareve and D.E. products is good intentions: with a pareve food, the line must be cleaned of dairy residue to the rabbi's satisfaction; whereas with a D.E. food, the line doesn't need to be so carefully cleaned, but no dairy products are included in the item's ingredients. Cookies, crackers, snacks, frozen desserts, and chocolate candies are all foods that are frequently processed on shared equipment. While a lactose-intolerant child, or even a child with a mild milk allergy, can most likely eat the food with no ill effect, a severely milk-allergic child may well have a reaction.

Kosher items marked *D* mean "dairy." That's a clear and simple warning to stay away.

So what's a parent to do? That most difficult of all things: use your best judgment. If your child has a history of anaphylactic reactions to milk, you should certainly avoid all foods marked *D* or *D.E.*, and be careful about the ones you choose that are marked *pareve*. Certain foods—chocolate, frozen desserts, and cookies—probably stand a higher chance of containing an unacceptable level of milk protein than, say, clear soups or pretzels. But that's not to say that the soups or pretzels can be absolutely, 100 percent guaranteed to not contain a speck of milk. The best you can do—the best *any* of us can do—is to make an informed choice, and be prepared to deal with the consequences if it turns out you've called it wrong.

WILL YOUR CHILD OUTGROW A MILK ALLERGY?

The odds are in your favor. Most children—about 85 percent—completely outgrow their milk allergies by the time they're three years old. And babies with enterocolitis generally outgrow their symptoms by the age of three as well.

Unfortunately, though, your milk-allergic little one is at a much higher risk for developing other food allergies. As reported by Dr. Sampson (in "Food Allergy," *JACI* [Journal of the Academy of Clinical Immunology], June 1999), 35 percent of infants with a milk allergy by one year of age had other food allergies by age three, and 25 percent had other food allergies by age ten. Because of this high correlation between milk allergy and other allergies, Dr. Sampson recommends that milk-allergic babies and toddlers be kept away from the allergens most likely to cause severe problems—eggs, peanuts, tree nuts, fish, and shellfish—before the age of three. The immune system seems to undergo a change at that point, with many children able to tolerate allergy-provoking foods without mounting an allergic reaction against them. Of course, you'll want to check with your child's health care professional before introducing any of these foods.

4

EGG

Allergies to egg are common in childhood and—happily—are frequently outgrown. But for the duration, complete and total avoidance not only is key to your child's health but greatly improves the odds that the allergy will be outgrown as soon as possible.

Total avoidance, of course, is easier said than done. Egg allergies are challenging on a number of levels. There's the "here, there, everywhere" problem of finding foods, particularly baked goods and desserts, that are completely egg-free. And there's the medical aspect: some vaccines—the influenza vaccine, for example—are cultured in egg protein. You'll want to consult both your pediatrician and your allergist on the best course to take when an egg-cultured vaccine seems in order.

Although for most children it's typically the egg white and not the yolk that contains the allergen, it's impossible to truly separate them so that not a speck of white remains. Don't even try. If and when your allergist decides that it's safe to challenge your child with egg, he or she will probably recommend that you begin with a small bite of yolk, knowing full well that some of the egg white will be present.

Egg Alert!

The following ingredients indicate the presence of egg protein and should be avoided by children allergic to eggs.

Albumin
Egg (white, yolk, dried, powdered, and egg solids)
Egg substitutes
Eggnog
Globulin
Livetin
Lysozyme (used in Europe)
Mayonnaise
Meringue
Ovalbumin
Ovomucin
Ovomucoid
Ovovitellin
Simplesse

Copyright © by the Food Allergy Network. Reprinted by permission of the Food Allergy Network.

Plenty of egg substitutes are available that will make baking quick, easy, and delicious. (These products are discussed later in this chapter and appear as ingredients in some of the recipes in chapter 16.) So please—stay away from the yolks.

Children who are allergic to egg *yolk* are also highly likely to be allergic to chicken, turkey, and other poultry.

There seems to be a strong correlation between egg allergy and asthma, with about 35 percent of egg-allergic children eventually developing the disease. Because asthma can also be triggered by environmental agents, you may want to think twice before installing wall-to-wall carpeting or getting a pet if your child is allergic to eggs.

But your main concern right now is just plain *eating*.

EGG-FREE BREAKFASTS

Some families, particularly those that include a child who is allergic to both milk *and* egg, find breakfast to be the most challenging meal of the day. Because my son Lucas is allergic to soy, egg, and milk, I used to worry that he wouldn't get any protein in his tummy until past noon. My solution was to treat breakfast like lunch and dinner. Lucas could have a ham sandwich with cut-up fruit for breakfast if he chose, or a bowl of pasta. In the winter, he might begin the day with a bowl of chicken soup. Other favorites included oatmeal—a nutritious grain that really sticks to kids' ribs—and a baked sweet potato with a little cinnamon and sugar. (The latter takes just four minutes to cook in the microwave at high power.)

When our family had a hankering for a "real" breakfast, I baked muffins or quick breads, made cinnamon toast with egg-free bread, or gave Lucas a bowl of cereal with Rice Dream. I added Rice Dream and egg-free substitute to pancake mix, too.

Not only Lucas but his older brother, Dylan, enjoyed the flexibility of being able to have dinner food for breakfast. As for me, I liked the fact that my boys were getting a good, nutritious start to the day.

ELIMINATING EGG FROM YOUR CHILD'S DIET

Let's begin with some practical guidelines:

• Avoid obvious egg sources: scrambled eggs, omelettes, timbales, souffles, custards, egg noodles, and eggnog. *Packaged egg substitutes are generally made with egg white and should be avoided.*

• A shiny glaze on baked goods is a signal that the food was probably brushed with egg before baking.

• Avoid mayonnaise and egg-based sauces such as hollandaise, béarnaise, Foyot, and Newburg. Salad dressings and sandwich spreads frequently contain egg as well.

• Assume that all bakery goods contain eggs. Some packaged cookies such as graham crackers and animal crackers may be egg-free, and some national brands of breads and crackers are egg-free, but be sure to check the labels carefully. When possible, bake your own egg-free cakes and cookies. (See chapter 16, "Recipes.")

• Avoid convenience foods and fast foods. All of the following may contain egg: canned goods, such as soups and pasta products; most packaged mixes for cakes, cookies, muffins, and pancakes; commercially prepared hot dogs and hamburgers; fried cheese sticks, chicken nuggets, and french fries; and, unfortunately, even pizza dough.

• Many ice creams, sherbets, sorbets, and other frozen desserts are made with egg. If you can't read the label, don't let your child eat them.

• Many popular candies contain egg, particularly egg whites. Read the labels carefully.

• Any meat that has been mixed with bread (such as meat loaf) or breaded (such as fried chicken) probably contains egg. Meats such as hot dogs, bologna, or sausages may include egg protein as an ingredient.

• Many pastas—not just egg noodles—contain egg. Read the labels carefully.

• Simplesse (fat substitute) contains egg protein.

• Do not use a pan that has been used to cook eggs unless you have first scrubbed it thoroughly with hot soap and water.

• Be sure to read chapter 12, "Hidden Allergens."

With these guidelines in mind, the easiest way to completely eliminate egg from your child's diet *and* keep everyone's sanity, especially for the purpose of a two-week trial elimination diet, is to keep it simple.

Eliminating egg is both harder and simpler than is seems: harder, because in baked or processed foods egg can show up just about anywhere; and simpler, because it's easy to get around. The key foods you need to identify and purchase are:

• Egg-free bread. (Many national brands are egg-free, both whole wheat and white.)

• Egg-free snack foods. (Most pretzels, chips, and gelatins, and many crackers, are egg-free. And of course, fresh fruits and veggies are the best snacks of all.)

• Egg-free desserts, if your family enjoys sweets. (Again, many national-brand ice creams, sorbets, puddings, and frozen treats are egg-free, but you must read each and every label. Stick to the brands that show the least number of polysyllabic ingredients.)

Eggs are an important source of B vitamins in a child's diet, but so are grains. If eggs are eliminated, you need to be sure that your child has a good source of whole grain products each day. Luckily, most children love breakfast cereal and sandwiches made with enriched bread—both excellent sources of B vitamins. Just check the label every time to make sure the products you've purchased are egg-free.

Most important, get R.E.A.L.: Read Every and All Labels!

If you're doing this elimination diet as part of a two-week trial run to see if eggs are the culprit in your child's allergic symptoms, it's best to stay away from restaurants, at least for these two weeks. There's simply too wide a margin for error. If your child is indeed diagnosed with an egg allergy or egg intolerance, you can refer to the many helpful strategies for eating out and traveling with egg allergies that are provided in chapter 21. But for now, keep the playing field completely clean.

EGG-FREE BAKING

Do you enjoy baking? It's hard to give up favorite foods, so now is a great time to give your child a pat on the back for being such a trouper. Two quick, delicious, and incredibly easy recipes I would recommend are the World's Best Chocolate Chip Cookies and Wacky Cake in chapter 16. Try them just once, and they'll become family favorites. Thanks to Rosemarie Emro's tireless efforts in her kitchen, a cookbook devoted solely to the topic of egg-free baking (titled, appropriately enough, *Bakin' without Eggs* and published by St. Martin's Press) even puts delicious egg-free cheesecake and brownies within easy reach. She and her publisher have kindly given me permission to include several of her wonderful recipes here (see chapter 16).

And remember to always look on the bright side: not only is baking without eggs easy, you have the added benefit of being able to freely sample the batter without fear of salmonella. So get out your teaspoons and dig into that cookie dough, and lick the chocolate cake spatula to your heart's delight.

5

WHEAT

Whether your child is diagnosed with a severe wheat allergy or simply garden-variety eczema caused by ingesting wheat products, one thing's for certain: you'll never look at a bagel or slice of bread in quite the same way again.

True wheat allergy is revealed through traditional allergy-testing techniques, that is, either a blood test or a skin test. Wheat-allergic children display the same range of symptoms as any other group of food-allergic children. Your child may have skin symptoms, respiratory symptoms, swelling of lips and tongue, intestinal symptoms, or a combination of these, ranging from mildly irritating to life threatening, depending on the severity of his or her allergy.

Although some people think that wheat allergy and gluten intolerance are one and the same, they are not. Gluten intolerance, also known as celiac sprue, is not a true allergy in the immunological sense, but rather a disease. With gluten intolerance, the proteins found in wheat, oats, rye, buckwheat, and barley irritate the lining of the small intestine, often severely. Because the small intestine is where most nutrient absorption takes place, children with untreated gluten intolerance do not receive adequate nutrition, even from a well-balanced diet.

Wheat Alert!

The following foods and ingredients indicate the presence of wheat and should be avoided by wheat-allergic children.

Bran
Bread crumbs
Bulgur
Cereal extract
Couscous
Cracker meal
Durum or durum flour
Enriched flour
Farina
Gluten
Graham flour
High gluten flour
High protein flour
Seitan
Semolina
Soft wheat flour
Spelt
Vital gluten
Wheat (bran, gluten, germ, malt, starch)
Whole wheat berries
Whole wheat flour

Other products that *may* include wheat protein include:

Gelatinized starch
Hydrolyzed vegetable protein
Modified food starch
Natural flavoring
Soy sauce
Starch
Vegetable gum
Vegetable starch

While milk, egg, peanut, and tree nut allergies pose a challenge to any parent's stress-management techniques and creativity, wheat allergies are in a class by themselves. They're not as common as the first four allergies, and they are frequently not as severe, but, according to mothers in the know, you don't know what frustration is until you've tried to make a wheat-free sandwich or bake a wheat-free cupcake that passes muster with a four-year-old. (I found my cupcake solution—Chocolate Dixies—quite by accident, when some icing I had prepared hardened inside a paper baking cup. See the recipe in chapter 16.)

Wheat and wheat products also have a nasty habit of turning up where we'd least expect to find them. Soy sauce, many canned soups, puddings, packaged shredded cheeses, and a wide variety of candies all contain wheat starch. Gravies and sauces—from béarnaise to barbecue—are generally thickened with flour. Even french fries are all too often coated with some form of wheat starch. In short, if your child is allergic to wheat, any processed food must be automatically suspect. (For a more complete rundown, see chapter 12, "Hidden Allergens.")

LIVING WHEAT-FREE—HAPPILY!

Wheat allergies demand that we turn our thinking around. If the answer to a problem isn't where we're looking for it, we must realize that it's where we're *not* looking for it. Once you've accepted that, everything gets a little easier. Knocking yourself out trying to make or buy a decent wheat-free pizza crust? Forget the crust; just grease a cookie sheet, pour some melted cheese into large circles or cookie-cutter shapes, bake for a few minutes, cool, remove, and top with tomato sauce. Running into the doldrums at breakfast time? Serve lunch or dinner foods instead. Stuff tuna or chicken salad into half a red pepper. Stir oatmeal or rice into meatballs. Learn how to bake meringues (or find a good commercially baked variety). Discover the joys of buckwheat (kasha), a satisfyingly chewy, nutty-tasting grain that is not related to wheat at all. It just takes a few tricks to make an extremely livable situation out of one that could appear near impossible.

It also helps to look to cuisines other than the standard American fare—heavy on refined flour—that most of us consider to be "our daily bread."

If wheat allergy is your sole concern, Asian food is a wonderful alternative, featuring bowls of delicious "sticky" rice and even rice noodles with every meal. (Be wary of the soy sauce, however; wheat is a hidden ingredient. And all dumplings, plus all other noodles *except* rice noodles and 100 percent buckwheat noodles, will contain wheat flour.)

My hands-down favorite for wheat-free "bread" is the Mexican corn tortilla. (Of course, be sure you read the ingredients or check with the chef to make sure that the tortilla your child will be eating is indeed made from 100 percent corn flour.) And some Indian food shops and restaurants offer breads made solely from lentil flour, known as papadum, that are every bit as satisfying as their wheat-based brethren. Of course, you will need to read the ingredients or ask the chef to make sure that *your* papadum is 100 percent wheat-free.

Although we usually think of Italian food and pasta as inseparable, Italian cooking has two major contributions to make to wheat-allergic people everywhere: risotto, an irresistible, slow-cooked rice dish; and polenta, a cornmeal dish. Both are popular with children in Italy, so there is no reason they shouldn't be popular with your little one here. Chapter 16 includes recipes for polenta and even a yummy polenta lasagna, as well as variations on a crustless "vegetable pie" that, when spread thin, makes an excellent alternative to pizza crust.

Health food stores across the country offer breads made from grains ranging from amaranth to rice to oatmeal to barley to spelt and kamut, which are ancient forms of wheat. Many wheat-allergic children can tolerate spelt and kamut, but many cannot, so don't serve either one before checking with your child's doctor. Quinoa is another grain that many wheat-allergic children can tolerate. If your child can eat spelt and quinoa, the pasta possibilities open up. You can buy spelt spaghetti, shells, and even elbows. And while spelt macaroni and cheese may fall short of the delicious casseroles of your youth, it's considerably better than none at all for your wheat-allergic child.

Health food stores are also a good source of frozen wheat-free waffles, wheat-free pancake, cookie, and cake mixes, and wheat-free crackers. A good number of these are quite good. You'll find wheat-free cookies, too, but for some reason most are unpalatable. Never mind; there are many delicious alternatives. Most health food stores also carry a nice variety of wheat-free flours and can give you tips on baking.

There are many books available on wheat allergies, some specifically for children. But my personal favorites are geared toward adults: *The Gluten-free Gourmet* books, by Bette Hagman, and *Against the Grain,* by Jax Peters Lowell. All are published by Henry Holt and Company.

GENERAL GUIDELINES FOR MANAGING YOUR CHILD'S WHEAT ALLERGY

The Food Allergy Network (FAN) often recommends the following wheat flour substitutes, which are each equivalent to one cup of wheat flour in baking.

- 1⅓ cups rice flour
- 1 cup barley flour
- ¾ cup amaranth flour plus ¼ cup either arrowroot, tapioca, or potato starch

1. Alternatives to wheat flour include rice flour, buckwheat flour (not in the same food family), potato starch, rye flour, oat flour, and barley flour. Products made from corn, amaranth, and quinoa may also be helpful. If you enjoy baking, stock some arrowroot, tapioca, or potato starch to blend with other flours. Health food stores and some mail-order companies are a wonderful source for alternative

wheat products. Be sure to check all cereal box labels carefully; some oat, corn, or rice cereals may contain whole wheat or wheat starch.

2. Avoid foods that contain malt or cereal extract, unless your child's doctor says that these foods are safe for your child to eat.

3. Be particularly careful around young children if adults are drinking beer, gin, or certain whiskeys. Although a young child should never "taste" an alcoholic beverage in the first place, accidents can happen. Taking a sip out of an unattended glass will be even more dangerous for a wheat-allergic kid.

4. Spelt and kamut, both ancient forms of wheat, *can* be less allergenic than wheat, depending on the severity of your child's allergy. They are not appropriate substitutes for everyone, however. Many breads, cereals, and mixes you may find in the health food store, touted as "wheat-free," will contain one or both of these products. It's important to check with your child's doctor before introducing your child to either spelt or kamut.

5. Beware of hidden allergens! Wheat and wheat products are frequently found in

- Baked goods and baked good mixes, including cakes, pies, cookies, crackers, muffins, and breads
- Chocolate and other candies
- Pancake and waffle mixes
- Sauces and gravies
- Processed meats, breaded meats, and meat casseroles
- Pastas
- Salad dressings
- Soups

See chapter 12, "Hidden Allergens," for a more thorough rundown of where wheat may hide.

6. Get R.E.A.L.! Read Every and All Labels!

6

PEANUT

Nuts grow on trees. Peanuts are *legumes,* growing on underground vines, extracting nitrogen from the soil to create a tasty, protein-rich seed. A prominent member of the pea family, the peanut is a kissing cousin of the lentil, garbanzo (chickpea), kidney bean, navy bean, pinto bean, black bean, soybean, and green bean. Originating in South America around 3000 B.C., peanuts have been an important food around the world for thousands of years. Today over 3 million Americans are allergic to peanuts, and the numbers are growing by leaps and bounds.

If your child is allergic to peanuts, you already know that peanut allergies are tough as can be. Reactions tend to come on almost immediately, are frequently severe, and should be considered life-long. Peanuts are composed of thirty-two different proteins, three of which have been implicated in causing an allergic reaction. This makes peanut such an extraordinarily powerful allergen that just smelling peanuts or an open jar of peanut butter can produce symptoms in some highly sensitive children—and many more will react to even the minute amount of peanut protein that is transferred when an imperfectly washed mixing bowl that held a peanut batter, for example, is used to prepare a batch of "peanut-free" cookies. To be more specific, *many peanut-allergic kids will react to the amount of peanut protein contained in less than* 1/100 *of a peanut.* Fortunately, more and more food manufacturers are now labeling foods that may have been exposed to peanut protein during the production process, particularly when foods are made on shared equipment.

The following ingredients indicate or may indicate the presence of peanuts in a food and should be avoided by children allergic to peanuts.

> Peanut (also watch for the line "may contain peanut traces")
> Cold-pressed or expeller-pressed peanut oil
> Ground nuts
> Mixed nuts
> Hydrolyzed vegetable protein (may contain peanut protein)
> Hydrolyzed plant protein
> Vegetable oil, if the vegetable is not specified (may be peanut oil)
> Peanut butter
> Peanut flour
> Peanut starch
> Beer nuts
> Artificial nuts (may be deflavored peanuts)
> Natural flavoring (may contain peanut protein)

Peanut allergies are especially tricky to deal with here in the United States because peanuts are all around us. In Scandinavia, where peanuts are eaten sparingly and rarely before the age of six, peanut allergy is virtually unheard-of. (As noted earlier, fish allergy is the big one there.) But we Americans consume *4 million pounds of peanuts daily,* spreading tablespoon after tablespoon of peanut butter on our bread, munching shelled peanuts by the handful in ballparks and bars, clamoring for more and more of them in our cookies, candies, muffins, and desserts.

What's more, peanuts turn up where you'd least expect to find them. Inexpensive, versatile, healthful (for most), and delicious, peanuts are ground to thicken soups, stews, veggie burgers, and casseroles, tossed in whole to add crunch to stir-frys and salads, and chopped to add rich texture to breads and sweet baked goods. In my own personal experience I've been astonished to discover peanuts or peanut oil in jelly beans, pizza, tomato sauce, vegetable soup, manicotti, and even pats of restaurant butter.

Forewarned Is Forearmed: Reducing the Risk of Peanut Allergy in Your Next Child

If you have one child with a peanut allergy, there's a good chance that other children you have will also be predisposed to developing a peanut allergy. But there are certain steps you can take before you even get pregnant to reduce the risk.

• Do not eat peanuts or peanut butter when you are trying to get pregnant, and avoid these foods completely once you become pregnant.

• Do not eat any peanut products while you are nursing. Peanut protein is passed through breast milk.

• Do not feed your younger child any foods with even trace amounts of peanut protein until the age of three.

• After your younger child reaches age three, consult your older child's health care professional about how you should proceed. If the doctor feels that a food challenge is in order, ask if you can do it in the doctor's office. Why deal with a reaction on your own if you don't have to?

In fact, experts say that one of the main reasons that peanut allergy has become so widespread is our widespread exposure to peanuts, beginning in utero. (Part of my own personal guilt trip is that during my pregnancy with Lucas, my daily 4 P.M. snack was an apple, sliced in eighths, lavished on every surface with my all-time swoon-food: Jif peanut butter. And I was certainly not above dipping a spoon in my own private jar, should the urge arise.) Peanut protein can also be found in breast milk. Given the growing number of moms who are breast-feeding (and no doubt enjoying peanuts, as most of us do), more and more children are being exposed to peanut protein in infancy—a time when the immune system is most likely to mount an allergic response.

What can be particularly frustrating to parents of peanut-allergic children is watching so many egg- and milk-allergic children grow out of their allergies, while peanut-allergic children generally do not. The very small exception to this rule seems to be children who had their first reaction, which was a *mild* anaphylactic reaction, before the age of two; had no subsequent reactions; and do not suffer from asthma. Of this group, a small percentage of children do appear to have outgrown their peanut allergy. If your child fits these criteria, you should consider having him or her retested for peanut allergy.

WHAT IS IT ABOUT PEANUTS THAT MAKES THEM SUCH POTENT ALLERGENS?

One theory is that the proteins found in peanuts (as well as tree nuts and shellfish) are extremely stable. Rather than being broken down as many proteins are in normal cooking and then in digestion, peanut protein remains whole and unchanged, impervious to heat, chewing, saliva, and stomach acid. So while a maturing immune system can learn to tolerate the relatively easy-to-break-down proteins found in

---

Peanut Allergy by the Numbers

- Five percent of children in the United States are allergic to peanuts.
- In just ten years, between 1984 and 1994, the amount of reported cases of peanut allergy doubled.
- It can take less than $\frac{1}{100}$ of a peanut to cause a life-threatening reaction.

milk and egg—hence the happy five-year-olds who can suddenly eat french toast and ice cream—peanut is simply too strong an opponent.

But that doesn't necessarily mean it's unbeatable. Dr. Hugh Sampson of the Elliot and Roslyn Jaffe Institute of Food Allergy at Mount Sinai Medical Center in New York City, who is currently working on an anti-IgE "vaccine" for peanut allergy (called the *safe shot*), shared an interesting tidbit of information with me at a recent meeting: while China is the world's leading producer of peanuts, and peanut products are used abundantly in Chinese cooking, peanut allergy is virtually unheard-of in China. Given the assumption that populations develop allergies based on how much they are exposed to a particular food, why aren't the Chinese more peanut-allergic?

One important distinction between the peanuts consumed in the United States and those consumed in China is that the Chinese peanuts are boiled, whereas the U.S. peanuts are roasted. Roasted peanuts typically reach a temperature of 245° C, whereas boiling occurs at 100° C. Proteins change in response to heat. Therefore, that higher temperature of the U.S. peanut may open the peanut protein in some way, making more allergy-producing material available to be bonded with. It's an intriguing theory.

There's no getting around it: when your child has a peanut allergy, assume nothing. That nice red lollipop being offered by the shoe salesman who just fitted your daughter with her fourth pair of sneakers this year? Pull a corresponding treat out of your bag and offer that one to her instead. That piping hot pizza at the birthday party, dripping with cheese and smelling divine? Call the pizzeria if you can, or just nuke the hamburger you brought. You get the idea. If you can't read the ingredients or confirm them with the chef, it's not meant to be.

When you dine out with a peanut-allergic child, it's better to steer clear of Chinese, Japanese, African, and Thai restaurants. Even if the restaurant does not cook with peanut oil, there are enough dishes with peanuts in them to make cross-contamination a likelihood rather than a possibility. If your child's Beef with Broccoli is prepared

Why Caution Is Key

A 1998 study of 122 peanut-allergic children showed that *56 percent experienced two cases of accidental ingestion over a 5.4-year period.* Most cases occurred outside the home.

in the same wok that just held Chicken in Peanut Sauce, be prepared to treat a reaction.

Ice cream shops are another peanut (and tree nut) allergy trap. You may very well have ordered a plain vanilla cone for your child and dutifully inquired about the ingredients. But where was the ice cream scoop last? Scooping out the Peanut Butter Fudge Ripple? And even if you ask the server to be sure to wash out the scoop, there is

Can Children "Outgrow" a Peanut Allergy?

The easy answer is, generally not. The more considered answer is, it depends. Occasionally a family may think a child has miraculously out-grown a peanut allergy when in fact the child was not allergic to peanuts in the first place.

Of the children who are truly allergic to peanuts, as confirmed by either a skin test or a blood test, the few who do indeed grow out of their allergy have these characteristics in common:

- Onset of peanut allergy early in life
- Fewer other allergies
- Fewer allergic symptoms such as asthma and eczema
- Smaller skin test (a hive that was a size 2 instead of a 4, for instance)

If your child meets these criteria, and has not had an allergic reaction to peanut in the past few years, retesting may be warranted. Under-stand, however, that these characteristics alone do not indicate that your child will outgrow a peanut allergy, or that you can be less vigilant. Outgrowing a peanut allergy is still the exception rather than the rule.

still a good chance that there are traces of unidentified ice cream in that vanilla barrel from all the other times a contaminated scoop passed through. The toppings are certain to hold mysterious items as well. And the same holds for milk-shake machines, unless you request that all parts be thoroughly washed before preparing your child's treat. It's best just to pass it all by.

But there is a light at the end of the tunnel. Many ice cream shops feature soft-serve ice cream or frozen yogurt as well, and most have a soft-serve machine that is *always* devoted to chocolate and vanilla. Ask and see if that is the case in your ice cream shop: after all, you wouldn't want to order soft-serve ice cream for your child out of a machine that just yesterday held Peanut Butter Cup Delight. If indeed that particular machine serves only chocolate and vanilla, and you have made sure that the ingredients for either flavor do not contain peanut, it would be highly unlikely for an accident to happen. This is exhausting, I know, but it does become second nature after a while.

PEANUT ALLERGY AND OTHER ALLERGIES

Some children who are allergic to peanuts will also have a positive skin test for one or more legumes, particularly soy. However, all legumes share a good number of proteins, making false positives a definite possibility. Unless your child has actually eaten a particular legume and experienced an allergic reaction, a positive scratch test *alone* is not proof that a true allergy exists. If your child is allergic to peanuts and everyone else in your family enjoys bean-based dishes, ask your allergist how to proceed. Each child is different, and every allergist has his or her own comfort level with food challenges, as does every family.

For many years, it was thought that there was no correlation between peanut allergies and allergies to tree nuts. Recently, however, the evidence seems to point to a link. Some major studies indicate that 35 percent of peanut-allergic children are also allergic to tree nuts, with Brazil nuts leading the pack as both the fastest-growing source of new allergies and the most severe. (In general, though, walnuts are the leading culprit in tree nut allergies.) Dr. Sampson reports seeing more seed allergies as well—sesame seeds, pumpkin seeds, poppy seeds, et cetera. So the moral of the story is: If you haven't yet introduced your peanut-allergic child to tree nuts, don't. If you have, it may not be a bad idea to phase them out of your child's diet, if only because tree nuts are generally processed on the same lines as peanuts, making the possibility for cross-contamination a very real issue.

Dr. Sampson also recommends keeping peanut-allergic kids away from shellfish and fish, as both of these foods are highly allergenic. When it comes to peanut allergy, discretion is most definitely the better part of valor.

Completely eliminating peanuts from your child's diet involves three steps:

1. Whenever possible, stick to whole, unprocessed, or minimally processed foods (fruits and vegetables, meats and eggs, milk and cheese, pasta and rice, and simple grain cereals). This makes good sense for all of us, but for peanut-allergic children it's particularly important. Eliminating or greatly reducing your child's intake of processed food has the added benefit of taking the worry out of eating—or at least reducing it considerably.

2. Get R.E.A.L.: Read Every and All Labels. No matter what the food, no matter how many times you've served it to your child, *read the ingredients label*. (And frankly, I read every ingredients label twice.) Ingredients may change at any time and may differ from region to region. Thirty seconds spent reading the label may very well save you the hours-long unpleasantness of a reaction or even a trip to the emergency room.

3. Whenever possible, bake it yourself. No, I'm not advocating rising at dawn to punch down the bread dough or roll out the biscuits. There are many national brands of breads and cookies you'll find safe to feed your child. But do yourself and your child a favor and stay away from bakeries. The possibilities for cross-contamination

are just too high. In chapter 16, I've included several cake and cookie recipes that everyone in the family will love, and they are quick and easy enough for even the most time-pressured parent to whip up.

THE PEANUT AND TREE NUT ALLERGY REGISTRY

Currently, over 4,000 children and adults in the United States and Canada are registered in two national studies supported by the Food Allergy Network. The purpose of the studies is to collect information to help researchers better understand the genetic basis of peanut allergy and how difficult it is to manage. Because peanut allergy is showing its greatest growth among children, the median age of the participants is five years. As of the time this book was written, 89 percent of the people registered had a reaction to peanuts, 265 also reacted to tree nuts, and 11 percent reacted only to tree nuts.

Information collected from the Peanut and Tree Nut Allergy Registry is being used to evaluate the circumstances under which reactions occur and what medications are being used to manage reactions. The registry is open to anyone with a peanut or tree nut allergy, whether or not that individual is a member of FAN and regardless of age. (So if your peanut-allergic child also has a peanut-allergic grandma, both of them can sign up.)

Researchers are also looking for twins (identical or fraternal) of any age to participate in a telephone questionnaire. One or both twins must have a peanut allergy. All information provided is kept strictly confidential.

To participate in one or both of the studies, call FAN at (800) 929-4040.

7

TREE NUTS AND SEEDS

Unlike peanuts, which belong to the legume family, tree nuts are true nuts—and among the most potent of all known food allergens. The tree nut family includes

- Almonds
- Brazil nuts
- Cashews
- Chestnuts
- Hazelnuts (also known as filberts)
- Hickory nuts
- Macadamia nuts
- Pecans
- Pine nuts (piñons)
- Pistachios
- Walnuts

While tree nut allergies have always been common in both children and adults, with walnut being the most common, recently doctors have been noticing an increase in the number and severity of allergic reactions relating to Brazil nut.

If your child is allergic to one kind of nut—almonds, let's say—it is not necessarily a done deal that he or she is allergic to *all* tree nuts. Only your doctor can run the appropriate tests and make that call. However, even if your child can safely eat other kinds of nuts, you still need to be very careful. And note that nut butters are almost always processed on the same equipment as are packaged nuts.

A new debate is opening up on whether children with severe nut allergy should avoid peanuts. (The highly peanut-allergic kids are now being told to stay away from all tree nuts before the age of three and to proceed with caution, if at all, after that.) A lot depends on the nature and severity of your child's allergy. Most doctors, however, noting that a child with a severe allergic reaction to tree nuts has already proved that he or she has the kind of immune system capable of severe allergic responses, will recommend that your child stay away from peanuts and peanut products at least until the age of three. The same goes for fish and shellfish—also highly allergenic foods. If your child has been happily eating peanut butter on toast and fish sticks since babyhood, however, there would probably be little reason to stop now.

Ingredient Terms You Should Know

Most of the time, reading a label in order to avoid nuts is fairly straight-forward. The label will clearly state *nuts, nut oil*, or the particular kind of nut or nut oil being used. Nut butters, too, are clearly marked and should be avoided. But nuts are also present when these terms are used:

- Almond extract
- Gianduja (chopped nuts mixed with chocolate)
- Marzipan (almond paste)
- Nu-Nuts artificial nuts
- Nut meal
- Mashuga nuts (pecans)
- Nougat
- Nut paste
- Piñon, pignoli (pine nuts)

©The Food Allergy Network

Are Water Chestnuts Safe for a Nut-Allergic Child?

Despite their name, water chestnuts are not nuts. They are corms—underwater roots. They are not related to nuts at all. (And as we've seen, peanuts are not nuts but legumes.) While children with serious nut allergies should avoid eating in Chinese restaurants due to the very high risk of cross-contamination, you shouldn't hesitate to whip up a stir-fry of your own at home, with a generous handful of these crunchy treats thrown in.

The bottom line is that only your child's doctor can make the final call. But do let discretion be the better part of valor, and consult the doctor before introducing any glamorous new foods to your nut-allergic little one.

As with all food allergies, complete and total avoidance of nuts is

Ranking the Nuts

When it comes to provoking an allergic response among people allergic to tree nuts, the top offenders, in order of prevalence, are:

1. Walnut
2. Almond
3. Cashew
4. Pecan
5. Hazelnut (filbert)
6. Brazil nut
7. Pistachio
8. Pine nut (piñon)
9. Other (may include chestnuts, macadamias, or hickory nuts)

This list is based on information provided by respondents to the Food Allergy Network's Peanut and Tree Nut Allergy Registry. Bear in mind that some people reported allergies to more than one kind of nut.

the only way to keep your nut-allergic child safe and healthy. Most very young children don't eat tree nuts whole—there's the danger of choking to contend with, for one thing—but it doesn't take much sleuthing to find them in foods children enjoy every day. Tree nuts are a popular addition to breakfast cereals and muffins, cookies and breads, ice cream treats and candies, waffles, snack foods, and crackers. I just may be paranoid (OK, I admit it, I am), but it does seem to me that every time a new variety of snack food is introduced, it seems to trumpet a "New, Nutty Taste!"

We're surrounded. In fact, by the time they're toddlers, most kids have had at least a tiny taste of tree nut in their lives, whether it was riding along in the bakery cookie Grandma bought or on top of the cereal flake that fell beneath the kitchen table. And once that initial exposure has occurred, the stage has been set for a possible allergic reaction the next time around.

Although nut allergies and peanut allergies are distinct, the same rules apply for avoiding them. The one bright note is that reading an ingredients label to avoid nuts is an easier task than it is for other foods. Simply avoid any food that has the name of a nut or the word *nut* anywhere on the label. Also be on the lookout for marzipan, nougat, and gianduja.

Commercial bakeries, even the finest, should be considered off-limits to a child with a serious tree nut allergy. There's just no way to clean the equipment thoroughly enough in between the walnut brownies, pecan sandies, or almond cookies, and your child's chocolate cupcake. Hygiene isn't the issue here—cross-contamination is. (If your child has a nut allergy, it is imperative that you read pages 128–130 in chapter 12, "Hidden Allergens.")

My friend Helen recently told me about buying a corn muffin for her daughter at a highly regarded local bakery. She asked the young lady behind the counter to check the ingredients and was assured that the corn muffin contained no nuts or peanuts. Her daughter took just one bite, spit it out, and said, "Mommy, this muffin has nuts in it." Within seconds, the little girl's lips began to swell with an allergic reaction, which Helen promptly treated. When Helen, at this point

---

Why You Can't Be Too Careful

When asked about the nature of their allergic reactions, the vast majority of respondents to the Food Allergy Network's Peanut and Tree Nut Allergy Registry reported urticaria (hives) upon their first exposure. About one in five reported wheezing or throat tightness, which can become life threatening. By the time of their third exposure, however, twice as many respondents experienced wheezing, and three times as many experienced throat tightness.

---

aghast, asked to speak personally to the baker, she found out that the corn muffin batter had been mixed in the same bowl as the banana-nut muffin batter—and hadn't been cleaned in between. Considering the high turnover in most bakeries, this practice is not at all uncommon. When it comes right down to it, all it takes is one dip of the wrong spatula into a non-nut batter to contaminate the whole batch. Who wants to take chances with that?

Candy shops that sell bulk chocolate and other confections by the pound are another potential minefield. Aside from everyday delights such as *nougat*—a nut-studded treat—and *marzipan*, which is made from almond paste, you may encounter exotic ingredients such as *gianduja*, a mixture of chocolate and chopped roasted nuts found in

---

Coffee Alert!

While few of us make a regular practice of giving young children sips of coffee, some kids do seem to relish the taste of it. If you enjoy coffee from gourmet coffee shops, bear in mind that your coffee may have been brewed in a carafe that just contained a nut-roast coffee. Enough cross-contamination can occur in these cases to cause a serious reaction.

---

many fine imported chocolates. And of course, there are always the mounds of cashew brittle, caramel-nut clusters, and pecan-studded fudge—piled right next to the sweet gummy bears you were thinking of buying for your child.

When you find yourself in a situation like this, you may feel that no one else really understands the potential danger to your child. But Dr. Hugh Sampson was recently delighted at the level of food-allergy awareness he encountered in one such candy shop in Chatham, Cape Cod. When asked if certain of the chocolates contained nuts, the young man behind the counter said that although they technically didn't, he knew that they had been stored with chocolates that definitely did, and so advised staying away from them. Not every counter person will be as forthcoming or as knowledgeable as this particular young man, but the point is well taken: unless the treat you want to give your child is well wrapped or in its own separate bag, the odds are high that it has had at least a chance encounter with something nutty during its life span.

Restaurants can also be a scary place for someone with nut allergies. Between the chicken salad with walnuts, the green beans with slivered almonds, and the pecan pie, there's more than one chance for a bit of cross-contamination to occur. Remember, also, that nuts are frequently chopped or ground and mixed into dishes where you'd least expect to find them.

We don't think of Italian food as using a lot of nuts, for example,

---

Chocolate You Can Feel Good About

Vermont Nut Free Chocolates is a mail-order company that was started by a mom with a nut-allergic child. The chocolates are gourmet-quality (but not gourmet-priced), come in many different varieties (including fun holiday shapes), are completely peanut- and nut-free, and are a hit with everyone we know. For more information, call (888) 4-NUT-FREE, or visit the company's Web site at www.vermontnutfree.com.

but pesto—chopped basil and pine nuts—could be in your child's ravioli or canneloni, in the sauce on your child's chicken, or even spread on the garlic bread. Nut oils can be used in cooking. Any time, in fact, that a food has a sauce or a filling—from barbecued ribs to stuffed chicken breast—there's the chance that a nut or two has found a tasty home. In general, the simpler the food, the safer it is. Consider ordering plain grilled or roasted meats, chicken, and vegetables; baked potatoes; simple pastas such as spaghetti with butter and cheese or a classic tomato sauce. But even the simplest dish can catch you unawares unless you've cleared it with the chef. *Always* tell your server about your child's food allergies when ordering, and be prepared with a safe choice if you don't feel satisfied with the answers you get from the kitchen staff.

SEEDS

I've included a section on seeds in this chapter because, like nuts, they are crunchy, high in protein, and show up almost everywhere. In recent years, they are also making a bigger name for themselves as allergy troublemakers, especially because they turn up where you'd least expect to find them. Sesame, poppy, and sunflower seeds are the chief offenders in this league. Mustard (yes, it's a seed) is particularly tricky; be especially wary of mayonnaise, prepared sandwiches and salads, marinades, salad dressings, grilled dishes, ground meat dishes such as meatballs and meat loaf, soups, stews, and gravies.

Pumpkin seeds are the only seeds that are fairly easy to avoid. (Mexican food is the one major exception—always ask about pumpkin seeds at a Mexican restaurant if your child is allergic to them.) If sesame or sunflower seeds are the problem, ask your child's doctor to tell you whether sesame or sunflower oil should be avoided as well. Many parents stay away from these oils, just to play it safe, but if your child's doctor says it's OK to use them, go ahead. Your life will be a lot easier.

As with nuts, baked goods are the favorite hiding place of seeds, followed closely by toppings, fillings, and sauces. Bagels or rolls tossed together in a basket, cookies piled together at the bakery, Chinese restaurants redolent of Sesame Beef—all should raise a red flag for you. The major problem with seeds, of course, is they're so darn small: it's easy to overlook that random sesame or poppy seed floating around in the fresh bag of rolls you just bought. Many national brands of breads contain sesame seeds or have been produced on lines with breads that do. In most cases, the manufacturer will state that on the label. Remember, Get R.E.A.L.: Read Every and All Labels!

8

SOYBEAN

The peanut's closest legume cousin—and virtually identical in protein structure—the humble soybean is a common cause of allergic reactions in babies and young children. The similarities stop there, however. Soy allergies are *usually* not life threatening (though in rare instances they can be) and, happily, are often outgrown, whereas peanut allergies should be considered lifelong. Pea and green bean are related allergies that may be present in childhood but are generally outgrown as well.

A quick word here about legumes in general: Many parents feel that if their child is allergic to soy or peanut, they should tread lightly around *all* legumes. After all, it would seem to make sense to stay away from foods that have so much in common—especially when the reactions can be so dramatic.

But once again, the world of food allergies confounds common sense. In the real world, an allergy to peanuts or soybeans rarely translates into an allergy to lentils, chickpeas (garbanzos), navy beans, kidney beans, black beans, pinto beans, or lima beans. And in

Watch Out for Soy!

The following is a partial list of ingredient terms that indicate the presence of soy.

- Hydrolyzed soy protein
- Miso
- Shoyu sauce
- Soy, including soy albumin, soy flour, soy grits, soy nuts, soy milk, or soy sprouts
- Soy protein, soy protein concentrate, or soy protein isolate
- Soy sauce
- Soybean, soybean granules, or soybean curd
- Tamari
- Tempeh
- Textured vegetable protein, also known as TVP
- Tofu

The following ingredients *may* indicate the presence of soy protein:

- Flavorings or natural flavoring
- Hydrolyzed plant protein
- Hydrolyzed vegetable protein
- Vegetable broth
- Vegetable gum
- Vegetable starch

the few cases where there does seem to be some sort of reaction going on, it's generally a mild one—a few hives, let's say.

In fact, many children who are allergic to soy can eat peanuts with no problem, and vice versa. What can be confusing is that because the two proteins are so similar, there is a high incidence of false positive scratch test results to soy in children who are allergic to peanut, and false positive scratch test results to peanut in children who are allergic to soy. Only your child's doctor can make the call in cases like that.

And of course, in the event of an anaphylactic reaction to *any* legume, you should always check with your child's doctor before introducing new foods in that family. Every individual has a unique immune system, and what's right for a hundred other kids may not be right for yours. Common sense also dictates that when you do introduce the new food, give just a bite or two the first time. That's a good practice for *anyone* with a food-allergic child.

Back to soy. Though we don't generally think of Americans as eating soy on a daily basis, and we certainly don't eat a lot of it, it's harder to eliminate from a child's diet than one would think. Soybeans and soy products, including soy flour and soy protein, show up in a wide range of popular, national-brand foods such as cereals, candy, crackers, margarine, cookies, hot cocoa mixes, canned soups, sauces, stews, and tuna, and enriched pastas and breads. (In fact, the very words *high protein*—usually so dear to parents' hearts—when used in relation to a grain product, should be a tip-off that soy flour is probably an ingredient.) Even many products that do not contain soy themselves—corn used in cereals, for example—are frequently processed with soybeans and so may contain traces of soy protein. In recent years food manufacturers have become much more enlightened about the dangers of cross-contamination, so in most cases you'll find the phrase "may contain soybean traces" in foods that may be affected.

In other words, if your child is allergic to soy, and his or her doctor has told you to avoid it altogether, you're not going to be a heavy consumer of processed foods—at least not most standard grocery store items.

The one bright spot is that the two major soy products used in what seems to be every processed food—soy oil and soy lecithin—are generally considered safe for children with soy allergies. As with all allergens, it's the protein that causes the reaction. In these two foods the protein is removed in their processing. Cold-pressed or expeller-pressed oils, on the other hand, may still retain enough of the protein to cause a problem. The oils will be listed like that on the label. If your child has a severe soy allergy, be sure to check.

9

FISH AND SHELLFISH

In terms of food families, fish and shellfish are not related. An allergy to one does not necessarily mean that your child will be allergic to the other. (Although a severe allergy to either should be taken as a strong warning to proceed with caution.) But the techniques for avoiding these foods are basically the same, so we've chosen to treat them as one category.

The bad news is, allergies to fish and shellfish tend to be severe and lifelong. The good news is, of all the common allergens, they are the most easily avoided—at least here in the United States.

Interestingly enough, in Scandinavia, where herring and other fish are a major part of the diet, fish allergy is prevalent, with an estimated 15 percent of the population affected. Spain and Italy show high incidences of fish and shellfish allergy too. But fish sticks and tuna fish sandwiches aside, we North Americans tend to think of fish and shellfish as more sophisticated grown-up fare, so it is possible that by not introducing our children to a wide variety of these foods at a young age we are offering them some protection.

Like an allergy to tree nuts, fish and shellfish are allergies that are often acquired in adulthood. It is not uncommon for someone who

---

Cross-Reactions

While it is not unheard-of for a child to be allergic to foods in three categories of seafood—let's say shrimp (shellfish), clams (bivalves), and tuna (fin fish)—in general a child will experience cross-reactivity within one particular group rather than across all groups. The exception may be with fin fish; for the most part, the fillet types of fish such as sole and flounder don't cross-react.

If your child is allergic to a food in one of the two categories below, it's best to avoid the entire food family. If your child has had an allergic reaction to one species of fin fish such as salmon or tuna, check with your doctor before introducing other fish.

Shellfish
Crabs
Crayfish
Lobster
Shrimp
Bivalves
Abalone
Clams
Conch
Mussels
Oysters
Scallops

---

had happily been eating shrimp, lobster, and crab for twenty or thirty years to suddenly experience a serious allergic reaction at an all-you-can-eat seafood buffet at the Maryland shore. Even the smell of shrimp, signifying shrimp protein in the air, can set off a reaction in a highly shrimp-allergic person. So if your child is highly allergic to fish or shellfish, you should probably not cook it at home. No wonder, then, that allergists urge parents of children with other food allergies to completely avoid introducing fish and shellfish until the children are at least three years old, and in the case of shellfish, cautiously if at all after that.

If your child has had an allergic reaction to one kind of fish—cod and salmon are common offenders here—you should steer clear of *all* fish. Happily, that's easy to do. Fish is seldom a "hidden" ingredient in foods—Worcestershire sauce, which has anchovies in it, being the major exception. (I did once read about someone having an allergic reaction to marshmallows—apparently the gelatin was made from fish bones—but it was an unusual case.) But it's always important to get R.E.A.L. and Read Every and All Labels for any processed or frozen foods you buy. You just never know.

Shellfish are even easier to avoid. If your child has had a reaction to any member of the shellfish family, you should avoid all shellfish. When it comes to premade foods, that's easy to do: because shellfish are considered *trayf*—not to be eaten—by people who observe the kosher dietary laws, you can be absolutely certain that frozen or canned foods marked *K* for "kosher" are shellfish-free.

Restaurants, as always, are another story. Don't take anything for granted. If your child's chicken or chop was broiled on the same surface as the Alaskan salmon—or fried in the same pan as the brook trout—you might run into some problems. Asian restaurants, which use a good deal of fish and shellfish, are probably best avoided. Shared woks and steamers are a fact of life in these establishments, and you don't want your child's health to be dependent on someone cleaning out a pan well enough. Also think twice about items that go into the deep-fat fryer, such as french fries, chicken nuggets, and fried cheese sticks. Are they cooked in the same hot oil as fish and shrimp? If your child's allergy is severe, the small amount of fish protein released into the oil upon cooking may be enough to trigger a reaction. Make sure the chef understands your child's special needs.

Remember that for many children, if an allergen even *touches* their food they will have a reaction. So that means no peeling the anchovies off a slice of pizza and giving it to your daughter, or letting her munch on the salad greens under your shrimp cocktail. And if *you* enjoy a lobster roll or eat fried shrimp or clams with your fingers, be sure to wash your hands with a moist towelette or *soap* and water before touching your son or his food. Water alone won't get the oils off.

Luckily, children with fish and shellfish allergies seldom feel deprived; birthday cakes, Halloween candy, and ice cream are blissfully allergen-free. Of course, if the highlight of your family's summer is a weeklong fishing trip, you might want to come up with an alternate plan—although "catch and release" is how many an avid angler plays the game, anyway. A few children are so exquisitely sensitive that even picking up shells at the beach can be a problem. If that is your situation, your warm-weather fun will have to center on a local swimming pool or artificial lake. But for the most part, if you exercise due caution in restaurants and other situations where cross-contamination may occur, your fish- or shellfish-allergic child can easily feel unhampered by his or her allergies, which is just the way it's supposed to be.

10

UNUSUAL ALLERGIES

Although the overwhelming majority of food allergies are caused by milk, eggs, wheat, soy, peanuts, tree nuts, fish, and shellfish, occasionally a child will react to other foods as well. As with any other food allergy, the reaction may be mild—a few hives or a minor bout of diarrhea, let's say—or as serious as anaphylaxis. And as with any other food allergy, once an unusual allergy is diagnosed, you must safeguard your child from eating the offending food.

This chapter is by no means an exhaustive treatment of all unusual allergies. Somebody, somewhere, at some time has probably been allergic to any given food on Earth. If you suspect your child is allergic to a particular food, no matter how odd or unusual it may seem (an allergy to rice, for example), you certainly should have it checked out by an allergist. Unusual does not mean impossible. The following allergies are unusual but are well documented.

Children who are allergic to *latex* will sometimes experience reactions to one or more of these foods, which are not in the same food family: banana, avocado, kiwi, chestnuts, and shrimp.

Some children, though by no means as many as people think, experience a reaction when they eat *strawberries*. Interestingly, strawberries naturally contain a good deal of histamine, the same chemical responsible for causing a lot of misery in allergic reactions.

Tomato allergy is also rare but problematic to manage out of the home. All soups, salads, gravies, casserole-type dishes, and chopped meat dishes must be considered suspect. Some children are allergic to both raw and cooked tomatoes, while others experience a reaction to tomatoes only when they are raw. *Potatoes*, which are also members of the nightshade family, can cause a skin reaction when they are handled raw, as in peeling.

In the legume family, *peas* and *lentils* are the biggest offenders after their notorious cousins, the peanut and the soybean. Both foods are easily avoided in American-style cooking but are a staple of Indian cuisine and vegetarian restaurants.

Very occasionally, a child will be allergic to *celery*, *garlic*, or *onions*. Celery is most associated with exercise-induced anaphylaxis, a condition that produces allergic symptoms only if the child engages in vigorous activity after eating.

Barley is a very unusual allergy that is primarily seen in babies who've just begun to eat barley cereal. Unfortunately, avoiding barley frequently means having to avoid most processed foods, as malt (made from barley) is found in the vast majority of them.

Allergies to *beef*, *pork*, and *chicken* are also very rare, but they do occur. Occasionally a child who is highly allergic to milk will have a beef allergy as well, and at other times the two will be unrelated. An allergy to egg yolk may predispose a child to an allergy to chicken, but it's possible to have the chicken allergy without the egg allergy. Children who are allergic to just one of these foods can simply omit it from their diet. If a child is allergic to two or all three, it's wise to consult a dietician to make sure the child is getting enough protein on a daily basis.

Very few children are allergic to *corn*, which is fortunate because some form of corn—such as cornstarch, cornmeal, baking powder, corn syrup, vegetable gum, modified food starch, and dextrose—is in virtually all manufactured and prepared foods. If your child is one of the rare kids with a true corn allergy, you may need to prepare all meals at home with known ingredients.

Melon and other *raw fruits* are primarily responsible for oral allergy syndrome, an uncomfortable but generally harmless itching in the mouth. Children with oral allergy syndrome will usually experience symptoms after eating only during certain seasons of the year. (See page 111.)

Again, if you suspect that your child is allergic to a particular food, do not let anyone tell you that it simply can't be true. Testing by an allergist is the only way to ascertain whether an allergy is present. While one would never wish a food allergy, unusual or otherwise, on a child, the only thing worse than dealing with a food allergy is ignoring one.

11

FOOD FAMILIES

If your child is allergic to one food, there's a chance that he or she will also be allergic to foods in the same family. The surprisingly tricky part is putting the foods and the families together. Peanuts, for example, are not a true nut. (Nuts grow on trees, while the peanut, a legume, grows on an underground vine.) Although it's not common, a percentage of peanut-allergic children are also allergic to the peanut's cousins: peas, green beans, soybeans, and all dried beans such as kidney and lentil. Because peanuts and tree nuts are not related, many peanut-allergic children can safely eat tree nuts (cashews, almonds, walnuts, pecans, pistachios, pine nuts, Brazil nuts, and macadamia nuts).

Still, it's not something we'd recommend. Tree nuts are a highly allergenic food in and of themselves, and recent studies have indicated a greater-than-average chance of a peanut-allergic child reacting to tree nuts as well. Tree nuts are also usually processed at a plant that processes peanuts as well. As any of you who have found a lone peanut in a jar of cashews can attest (it's happened to me at least a dozen times), the possibilities for cross-contamination are very high. Any severely peanut-allergic child is probably best off trying tree nuts

---

Food Family Facts

- Eleven percent of people with food allergies react to more than one food.
- Five percent of people with legume allergy react to more than one legume.
- Fifteen percent of people with grain allergy react to more than one grain.
- Fifteen to 40 percent of people with tree nut allergies react to more than one tree nut.
- Thirty to 100 percent of people with fish allergies react to more than one fish.

---

for the first time, if at all, in a controlled food challenge at your allergist's office. (Read about food challenges in chapter 1.)

What's more, bear in mind that cashew and almond butter are almost always processed on the same equipment used to process peanut butter. Sticky, gooey nut butters are very difficult to clean out of machinery, so the chance of some dangerous cross-contamination occurring is very real.

THE MOST COMMON PLANT AND ANIMAL FAMILIES

Buckwheat	Buckwheat, rhubarb
Cashew	Cashew nut, mango, pistachio
Citrus	Grapefruit, lemon, lime, orange, tangerine
Fungi	Mushroom, yeast
Ginger	Cardamom, ginger, turmeric
Goosefoot	Beet, spinach, Swiss chard
Gourd	Cantaloupe, cucumber, pumpkin, squash, watermelon

Grass (grains)	Bamboo shoots, barley, brown cane sugar, corn, kamut, millet, molasses, rye, sorghum, spelt, wheat, wild rice
Heath	Blueberry, cranberry
Kola nut	Chocolate (cocoa), cola
Laurel	Avocado, bay leaf, cinnamon, sassafras
Lily	Asparagus, chives, garlic, leek, onion, sarsaparilla
Mallow	Cottonseed, okra
Mint	Balm, basil, bergamot, hoarhound, marjoram, oregano, peppermint, rosemary, sage, savory, spearmint, thyme
Mustard	Broccoli, brussels sprouts, cabbage, cauliflower, Chinese cabbage, collards, horseradish, kale, kohlrabi, mustard, radish, rutabaga, turnip, watercress
Myrtle	Allspice, clove, guava
Nightshade	Bell pepper, cayenne, chili pepper, eggplant, paprika, pimiento, potato, red pepper, tobacco, tomato
Palm	Coconut, date
Parsley	Angelica, anise, caraway seed, carrot, celery, celery seed, coriander, cumin, lovage, parsnip, samphire, sweet Cicely
Pea (legume)	Acacia, black-eyed pea, dry beans, green bean, lentils, licorice, pea, peanut, soybean
Plum	Almond, apricot, cherry, nectarine, peach, plum and prune
Rose	Blackberry, raspberry, strawberry, all other bramble berries

Sunflower	Artichoke, chicory, dandelion, endive, lettuce, salsify, sunflower seed, tarragon (ragweed and pyrethrum are related inhalants)
Walnut	Butternut, hickory nut, pecan, walnut
Plant foods without relatives (These foods are not related to one another or to any other foods.)	Arrowroot, banana, black and white pepper, Brazil nut, chestnut, chicle, coffee, elderberry, fig, flaxseed, gooseberry and currant, grape and raisin, hazelnut, honey, karaya gum, macadamia nut, maple sugar, New Zealand spinach, nutmeg and mace, olive, papaya, persimmon, pineapple, poppy seed, sesame seed, sweet potato, tapioca, tea, vanilla
Mollusks	Abalone, clam, oyster
Crayfish	Crab, lobster, prawns, shrimp
Fish	All true fish such as catfish, perch, salmon, tuna
Birds	Chicken, duck, egg, goose, pheasant, quail, turkey
Mammals	Beef, cow's milk, goat's milk, lamb, pork, rabbit, squirrel, venison
Chemicals and drugs	Antibiotics, aspirin, barbiturates, flavors, food color, fruit acids, sulfa drugs, sweeteners, tranquilizers, other drugs

INTERACTIONS BETWEEN FOOD AND NONFOOD FAMILIES: ORAL ALLERGY SYNDROME

Although allergies to fresh fruits and vegetables are relatively rare, occasionally a child will experience what is known as oral allergy syndrome when eating certain fruits and vegetables that cross-react with some of the pollens that cause hay fever.

Oral allergy syndrome is uncomfortable but generally not serious. Children may experience an itchy and/or tingling sensation in their mouths, tongue, palate, and throat that may feel as if it's spreading to the ear. There may be some edema (swelling) of the lips, tongue, and/or palate, and a feeling of throat tightness. The symptoms can be alarming, but they don't usually progress to any other body systems. A dose of antihistamine is all that's required in most cases. However—if your child ever experiences a food-related episode of swelling and throat tightness, let your *doctor* decide if oral allergy syndrome is the cause.

The table below shows the most common offenders and the pollen causing the cross-reaction (pollenosis).

BIRCH	RAGWEED	GRASS
Apple	Banana	Cherry
Carrot	Cantaloupe	Peach
Celery	Honeydew	Potato
Hazelnut	Watermelon	Tomato
Kiwi		
Potato		

Your child may experience symptoms when eating these *fresh* fruits and vegetables (but not when they are cooked):

- Apples, citrus fruits, pears
- Apricots, cherries, peaches, plums
- Broccoli, carrots, celery, tomato

Once diagnosed, oral allergy syndrome is managed the same way as any food allergy: avoid the trigger foods (in this case the raw forms of the foods listed), carry antihistamine in case of accidental ingestion, and educate both your child and any caregivers on what symptoms to watch out for and how to treat them.

12

HIDDEN ALLERGENS

Every time your child eats a food that is not in its whole, unprocessed state—potato chips, for example, instead of a plain baked potato; or chocolate chip ice cream instead of a glass of milk—there is a small yet real possibility that some "hidden allergens" are coming along for the ride. That's just the price we pay for living in the modern world with its complex means of food production and its ever-more-complex food supply.

Sometimes these allergens are not really hidden—they're right there on the label. It's just you'd never expect to find them and wouldn't necessarily think to look or ask, although you always should. Shredded cheeses, for example, frequently have flour added to prevent caking. Soy sauce is made with wheat. Baking powder usually has cornstarch as an ingredient, and vanilla extract may contain corn syrup. Soy flour is an ingredient in many enriched breads. Potato chips may be fried in peanut oil.

Carefully reading the ingredients is crucial to staying safe with food allergies. But it's not always enough.

For example: Let's say you just bought a package of granola bars for your allergic son. You've read the label three times and found no trace of food or additive that could be linked to his allergy. Are the granola bars safe for him to eat?

It's hard to say. Major food manufacturers in the United States, who were as a rule responsible to begin with, have in recent years become much clearer and more vigilant in their labeling. This is thanks in no small part to the efforts of the Food Allergy Network. Since 1994, when I first began seriously reading ingredient labels, I have seen a major difference in the way ingredients are listed.

Some manufacturers now print common allergens such as milk, eggs, wheat, corn, soy, peanut, and nut in bold type on their labels, and state the allergens again below the ingredients list. Others alert consumers to the fact that some cross-contamination may have occurred with ingredients. Plain M&M's, for example, list peanut on their ingredients because they are processed on the same equipment as peanut M&M's. Some corn cereals warn that the corn was processed with soybeans and thus may contain trace amounts of soy.

Careful labeling is all well and good, but it *doesn't* eliminate the

---

To keep your food-allergic child safe you must read every label! Often the information you need most is at the very end of the ingredients list or in fine print.

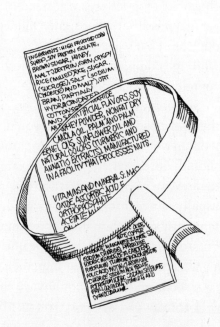

need for a judgment call on your part. Think about those granola bars. Are there varieties made by the same manufacturer that *do* contain foods your son shouldn't eat? A nut variety of granola bar, or a frosted variety that may contain milk or egg? If so, there is a possibility of cross-contamination and even the remote chance that your package will contain the wrong kind of granola bars. (Mix-ups like this are rare, but they do happen.)

Label Alert 101

There is no denying that labeling practices by major food manufacturers have improved significantly over the past five years. However, we still have quite a way to go before food labels are clear and easy for *everybody*—not just well-educated parents and professionals—to read.

The bogeymen to look out for are:

- The many (and often esoteric) words used to denote a single food allergen. *Example:* lactose, whey, casein, and caramel color can all indicate the presence of milk protein.
- "Misleading" labeling. *Example:* some "nondairy" foods do in fact contain milk protein (such as soy or lactose-free cheeses, or sorbets that are made on dairy equipment).
- Ingredient switching. *Example:* almonds were too expensive to be added to the cookie mix, so pecans were put in instead.
- "Hydrolyzed" protein and "natural" flavoring, which can contain protein from major allergens.
- Outsourcing components. *Example:* the cocoa used in "milk-free" chocolate was produced at the same plant as milk-containing hot cocoa mix.
- Contamination from production equipment, packing equipment, or wrappers.

Is an ingredient listed—margarine, for example—that is really made up of several ingredients without those ingredients listed separately? Margarine can contain milk or soy, triggering a reaction in your child.

Many manufacturers do break down complex ingredients, listing the components in parentheses on their labels, but many do not. I have seen "pasta product" listed as an ingredient in rice mixes (there's definitely wheat and possibly egg hiding in there), as well as "vegetable oil" with no explanation of which vegetable that might be (peanut, soy, sunflower, sesame, and nut oils can all fall under the umbrella of "vegetable oil").

And sometimes, important ingredients are left off the label altogether, despite extensive proofreading and the manufacturer's best intentions. We are humans, after all, and humans make mistakes. I receive, on average, two mailings a month from the Food Allergy Network, alerting its members to a mislabeled product containing potentially dangerous allergens—usually milk, egg, peanut, tree nut, or wheat. The product is always recalled as soon as the mislabeling becomes apparent, and the manufacturers themselves often fund the mailing. The intentions are good on all sides. But the simple fact remains that mistakes sometimes happen.

Another form of "hidden allergen" is the "secret ingredient" many restaurants add to their foods. An often-quoted example is the nineteen-year-old Brown University student who knew she was allergic to peanuts. She died in a restaurant after eating just a few teaspoons of a bowl of chili—chili made with peanut butter. Recently, another peanut-allergic young girl became seriously ill after eating a pasta dish at an Italian restaurant that had peanuts as a hidden ingredient. It's quite possible that both of these incidents would have been avoided had someone asked the restaurant staff about the ingredients in each dish. But who in a million years would expect to find peanuts in chili or manicotti?

Unfortunately, in the world of food allergy, you can't take anything, no matter how seemingly obvious, for granted. I have found peanut oil listed as an ingredient in jelly beans (jelly beans!), vegetable soup, and tomato paste, not to mention the more plausible uses in baked goods and chips. When we went to Walt Disney World in 1998, at least half of the restaurants we visited cooked their french fries in peanut oil, and many included egg in their pizza dough. And recently, a friend called to let me know that a neighborhood pizza restaurant uses peanut oil in its pizzas.

What can you, as a parent, do?

For starters, you need to determine how much risk you're willing to live with in exchange for the convenience and fun of dining out or eating prepackaged foods. Manufacturers do make every effort to label foods properly, and most restaurants, when alerted, are careful and responsible. However, they are *not* required by law to alert consumers to possible cross-contamination. And sometimes, albeit rarely, major accidents do happen. Peanut butter gets into the cheese crackers or vice versa. Egg whites are inadvertently left off the label. You simply have to decide if you want to take any risks at all.

To a certain degree, your decision will depend on what your child's allergies are, as well as their severity. If your daughter is extremely allergic to milk and eggs, for example, you'll have to be a lot more careful about selecting packaged baked goods than the parent of a child with a shellfish allergy. Or if your son is allergic to some nuts, you'll probably want to skip *all* nut butters, but will most likely feel reasonably safe about allowing him to eat commercially produced breads (after you've read the ingredients, of course).

It all boils down to a matter of common sense plus how trusting you feel on any given day.

You also need to consider the source. Local markets and even regional chains that put their own labels on breads and baked goods prepared on the premises are probably not paying the same attention

---

Latex Alert!

If your child is allergic to latex, you should know that there have been some reported cases of latex reactions occurring in restaurants where food workers wear latex gloves. If the worker stirs a drink with a gloved finger or handles a lot of food with gloved hands, enough latex may be transferred to the food to cause an allergic reaction.

to quality control as major food manufacturers. Those labels are just printed up and pasted on. I've seen mislabeled items too often to count—nuts in chocolate chip cookies, bran muffins sold in a corn muffins box, whole wheat baguettes in a sourdough wrapper. This isn't to say that the products aren't fresh, wholesome, and delicious. Quite often, they are. There's also a good chance that they're not exactly as represented.

Likewise, if your child has a peanut or nut allergy, it's probably best to proceed with extreme caution when buying treats from a bakery. (If the allergy is to milk or eggs, I recommend that you do your own baking at home.) For one thing, it's simply not practical for bakeries to break down and thoroughly clean every single piece of equipment in between recipes. For the relatively small amount of goods produced, it just isn't worth it. But if your child's chocolate birthday cake was run in the mixer right after the nut bread or peanut butter cupcakes, there's a real risk of cross-contamination.

Another variable in bakeries is the personnel. In a restaurant, a waitress can run into the kitchen and quiz the chef on the exact ingredients in your child's meal. In a bakery, the baker may not even be on the premises anymore by the time you make your purchase. You're relying on the knowledge of the counter person, who may or may not know exactly what goes into the cake, cookies, and pie. (And who would most definitely not know if there was an opportunity for cross-contamination to occur.)

Nut cross-contamination can be a real problem at the ice cream parlor. Unless the server thoroughly cleans the ice cream scoop before serving your nut-allergic child (or thoroughly washes out the milkshake machine), there's a good chance that a smidgen of butter pecan or almond fudge or peanut butter ice cream will be coming along for the ride on your child's cone (or in the shake). With soft-serve treats, it's wise to ask if a nut-containing variety was in the machine in the past few days. If it was, stay away.

If your child is highly allergic to dairy, beware the deli counter. That yummy ham or turkey you just ordered may have been sliced right after an order of cheese. Naturally, some cheese will be left on the blade, and chances are good that some of it will end up in your order as well. (Just because you can't see it doesn't mean it isn't there and capable of causing a reaction.) The same holds true at the salad bar: the tongs you are using to create an allergen-free salad may have just held shredded cheese or a salad containing milk products.

When eating in restaurants, it's best either to bring a safe meal with you or order the simplest meal possible: plain grilled meat or chicken, baked potato, and salad or vegetable. Be sure to ask about cooking oils, marinades, butter, or margarine that may be brushed on the grilled meat. Anytime you are dealing with more than one ingredient, keep your antennae up. If your child loves hamburgers, you'll have to find out if the patties are 100 percent beef—there could be soy, wheat, even egg or other fillers hiding in there. If the allergy is to milk, egg, soy, wheat, peanut, or nuts, bring your own dessert. We bring our own milk- and egg-free hamburger buns and home-baked cookies to local restaurants. And frankly, we don't eat out as much as we used to.

Most important, we all need to get R.E.A.L.: Read Every and All Labels. No matter if your child has had the same breakfast cereal every morning of his or her life, before you open a new box, read the ingredients. Every carton of crackers, every loaf of bread, every box of pasta, every package of cookies: *READ THE LABEL.* Even tried-and-true formulations for breakfast sausage, canned tuna, or frozen waffles can suddenly contain new ingredients. What's more, the ingredients can and do change without warning anywhere else on the box. Get R.E.A.L. Read the label. It just takes a few seconds to prevent a reaction.

I make this next suggestion with all due love and respect to those of you who are not particularly happy in the kitchen: you might want to pull a few good recipes together, dig up some pots and pans, and do some cooking.

Now I am a person who used to believe that life without takeout was basically not worth living. When I was invited to a friend's "Bring Your Favorite Recipe" bridal shower, my contribution was an index card detailing how to order Chinese food over the phone. (Step 1. Select menu from generous assortment on front hall desk.)

My mother made sure that I had basic cooking survival skills plus a few "company dishes," but my life plan was that I'd never reach the point where I'd actually have to use them—at least not on a regular basis. So if you're reading this section and just hating every word of it, I truly understand. On the other hand, I would just as soon spare you the pain of an emergency room visit. None of the recipes I've included in chapter 16 are difficult, and all have been enjoyed by my family for many years. Give them a try.

The long and short of it is this: unless a food is whole and unprocessed—or prepared from unprocessed foods by your own two hands—there is the chance that something you don't know about or want is in there. It's like the new airport security, where you're asked to vouch that you packed your own luggage, you've been watching it the whole time, and no one asked you to carry anything on for them. In both cases—with food allergies and on the airplane—you have to watch out for bombs.

What follows is a case-by-case survey of where hidden—or surprising—allergens may be found. Although it is thorough, no survey like this can ever be considered complete. (Life in the food-allergy universe is never that simple.) Use it as a guide to avoid common causes of accidental exposure, but exercise your own judgment—and ask when in doubt.

MILK

At the deli counter:

If your child is highly allergic to milk, remember that deli slicing equipment is used for cheeses as well as meats. It is highly likely that some cross-contamination will occur at any given time, and inevitable that cross-contamination will occur if the order or two before yours was for sliced cheese. The only way to completely guarantee your child's safety is to purchase prepackaged kosher deli meats, as kosher dietary laws prohibit mixing milk with meat. If you have the great good fortune to live near a kosher deli, by all means buy your fresh sliced meats from there.

Other sources of potential milk reactions at the deli counter include:

- Caramel color (may contain milk protein), found in many deli meats
- Natural flavor (may contain milk protein), found in many deli meats
- Milk or milk products in nonkosher meats such as frankfurters, bologna, salami, and other sausages
- Any deli salads, due to the possibility of cross-contamination with milk-containing side dishes such as coleslaw and macaroni salad
- Sandwich breads and rolls (may contain milk)

At ice cream and candy stores:

While it's obvious that milk can be found in ice cream, frozen yogurt, sherbets, and most varieties of chocolate, it can lurk in virtually any confection, including hard candies, jelly beans, and candy corn. Do not allow your child to eat any candy or frozen treat unless you can read the ingredients, and watch out for the following situations.

- Milk-free chocolates or candies may be stored or displayed alongside milk-containing varieties. If the candies touch, or if the same scoop is used to serve them, there may be enough milk protein exchanged to give your child a reaction. Your safest bets are labeled, individually wrapped chocolate bars or labeled bags of candy.
- Read labels with extra care; a chocolate bar or bag of candy may not list milk on the ingredients but may be marked *D* (dairy) or *D.E.* (dairy equipment), which means the sweet was processed on the same line as a milk-containing product.
- Some ice cream shops sell soft frozen fruit treats that are advertised as milk-free. Skepticism is the safest route here: just saying it's so doesn't make it so. There may be casein (a milk protein) or natural flavor that contains milk protein in the product. Ask to read an ingredients statement. A safer bet (though not always an option) may be to purchase an individually wrapped and labeled popsicle or similar frozen confection.

• Sorbets may very well be milk-free (ask to read the ingredients), but if they are being scooped out of a barrel in an ice cream shop, they have invariably been contaminated with milk protein. Avoid them.

In restaurants:

• Butter is a restaurant's favorite ingredient because it makes things taste so good. Some well-known chefs confess to adding a stick or more of butter to a single entree. Even when exercising more restraint, many restaurant chefs believe that brushing butter on a broiling steak, slathering butter over roasted chicken, and adding a fat pat of butter to vegetables is all in the name of gustatory pleasure. Unfortunately, however, when you inquire about a milk allergy, not everyone will make the butter connection. Be specific and crystal clear that your child's meal must be absolutely plain.

• Avoid salad bars and family-style buffets at all costs. Cross-contamination of the food is virtually guaranteed.

• Frying oils are notorious carriers of allergens. If the restaurant features fried chicken or fish (which are often dipped in milk before coating), fried mozzarella sticks, or any other milk-containing fried food, it would probably be best for your child to avoid eating the restaurant's french fries unless they are cooked in a separate fryer. Be sure to ask if the french fries have a coating that contains milk, as many do.

• Breads, bread sticks, and crackers may be baked with butter or other milk products.

• Tomato sauces are frequently made with cheese or other milk products.

• Salad dressings, apart from plain oil and vinegar, may have cheese, whey, or other milk protein in them.

• Soups, stews, and meat gravies are often thickened with a roux made from browned butter and flour. Even if the item in question is a plain vegetable broth, ask specifically if it contains milk or butter. Better yet, avoid soups and gravies altogether.

• In fact, it's probably safest to assume that any casserole dish—

from chili to pasta dishes—has at least some milk protein in it. Stick to single-ingredient entrees.

• Desserts other than fresh fruit are a risky proposition. If your family enjoys restaurant desserts, pack a safe baked treat or milk-free chocolate bar for your child.

At the grocery store:

• Remember that *lactose-free* and *dairy-free* do not usually mean free of all milk protein. Soy and "veggie" cheeses contain casein, a milk protein, and some may even contain whey. Dairy-free frozen desserts may be processed on a line with dairy products, which should be noted on or directly below the ingredients list.

• Avoid the in-store salad bar. Cross-contamination is a given.

• Most brands of margarine contain milk.

• Packaged foods—including the breads, pretzels, crackers, cereals, candies, and cookies that you've regularly bought for years—can change ingredients at any time. Be sure to get R.E.A.L. and Read Every and All Labels—*every time.*

• "Fun size" versions of candy may contain different ingredients than the regular-size products.

• Fat-free or low-fat versions of products you regularly use will have different ingredients.

• Strange as it may seem, even canned meats and fish may contain milk protein.

Miscellaneous:

• Milk protein may be present in prescription and over-the-counter medications. Always read the label or consult the *Physician's Desk Reference* before giving your child medication.

• Food for dogs and cats frequently contains milk protein. Keep your little one away from the pet food dish!

• Many personal care products such as lotions, soaps, and shampoos are made with milk or milk protein.

EGGS

At the deli counter:

• Because mayonnaise is rich in eggs, and deli salads are rich in mayonnaise, avoid giving your child *any* salad item from the deli department. With different shifts of workers serving hundreds of customers each day, the odds are great that someone will stick the wrong spoon into the wrong bin and introduce egg protein, let's say, into the Greek olives or fruit salad.

• Because many pastas have egg in the recipe, avoid pasta salads.

• Many breads and rolls are made with egg. If you would like your child to have a sandwich prepared with deli meats, buy a bag of rolls that have the ingredients listed and ask the counter person to slice the meat onto one of them.

• Prepared hot items—such as knishes, pizzas, fried chicken, macaroni and cheese, meatballs, and soups—may contain egg protein and should be avoided.

At ice cream and candy stores:

• Many ice creams, particularly premium brands, get their richness from eggs. So do many frozen yogurts, fine sherbets, and sorbets. Always ask about the ingredients. If one flavor is made with egg, you must assume that the other barrels of ice cream have been cross-contaminated. Soft-serve treats—provided the ingredients check out—are a safer bet.

• Egg protein may be an ingredient in sprinkles and other toppings.

• Many candies are made with egg. If the same serving scoop is used for a variety of candies, you must assume some cross-contamination has occurred. Prepackaged or individually wrapped candies are a safer choice.

In restaurants:

• Deep dish pizzas often incorporate egg in the dough, and other pizzas may as well. Always ask.

• Avoid the salad bar and family-style buffets at all costs. Cross-contamination is virtually guaranteed.

• Many pastas are made with egg.

• Any ground meat dish—lasagna, meat loaf, meat-filled dumplings, or meatballs, for example—will probably have some egg in it.

• Fried foods, including french fries, frequently have an egg coating. Any dish that requires one of its elements to be fried before being added to the casserole—eggplant parmigiana, for instance—may be made with egg.

• Any breaded item probably includes egg in the recipe.

• Soups, particularly those with pasta or meatballs in them, frequently use egg protein.

• Salad dressings, apart from plain oil and vinegar, often contain eggs.

• Because many breads are baked with egg, avoid the bread basket and hamburger bun.

• Many Chinese dishes—from fried rice to egg rolls, egg foo young, egg drop soup, and others—are heavily laden with egg.

• Milk shakes may be made with egg-laden ice cream. There may be egg protein in smoothies as well.

At the grocery store:

• Many ice creams and frozen desserts, including sherbets, sorbets, and others, are manufactured with egg ingredients. Get R.E.A.L.: Read Every and All Labels.

• Any baked goods—such as breads, crackers, cookies, bagels, rolls, cakes, donuts, and muffins—usually have egg in the recipe. If you cannot read the label, do not allow your child to eat it.

• Frozen waffles and pancakes are almost always made with eggs.

• Many candies, including candy corn, jelly beans, chocolate, and chocolate mints, may hide egg protein. Always read the label.

• Canned soups are another place where egg protein may be hidden.

• Granola bars and similar products may include egg as an ingredient.

PEANUTS

At *the deli counter*:

• Peanuts may be added to deli salads or used as a thickening agent in hot dishes.

• Fried foods and roasted chickens may contain peanut oil.

• If peanut butter sandwiches are made at the deli counter, the knives and counters probably have enough peanut protein on them to cause a reaction. Ask for a few ounces of sliced meat or cheese wrapped in paper, and make your child's sandwich yourself.

At *ice cream and candy stores*:

• Peanuts, peanut starch, or peanut oil may be in any candy at all. If a peanut-free candy is stored with candy containing peanuts, the peanut-free candy must be considered unsafe to eat. Only allow your child to eat wrapped candy with an ingredients label that you can read.

• Ice cream shops use the same scoops for all ice cream flavors, so cross-contamination is a given. If possible, order your child a soft-serve cone, after you have determined that no peanuts are in the flavor and no peanut flavor has been served from that machine for a few days at least.

At the grocery store:

- Many cereals either contain peanuts or are processed on the same line with peanut-containing products. Always read the label.
- Many crackers are processed on the same line as peanut-filled varieties. Read the label.
- Breads and muffins may contain peanuts or peanut flour, or may be processed on the same line with those that do.
- Do not allow your child to eat cookies, cupcakes, donuts, muffins, or other treats displayed in a bakery case. Not only are the ingredients a mystery, there is a good chance that even a "safe" item will have rubbed shoulders with a peanut-containing one.
- Avoid store-packaged bakery items, even those with ingredients labels. It has been my experience that these are less than reliable.
- Carefully read the labels on all packaged candies, including chocolate chips. It seems that the majority these days will say "may contain peanut traces."
- Use your own judgment with granola bars and granola cereals. Personally, I avoid them at all costs.

In restaurants:

- Any fried foods—from chicken to french fries to potato chips—may have been fried in peanut oil. If the chef tells you the oil is a blended vegetable oil, it may contain peanut oil. If the oil itself is safe, but if foods containing peanuts are then fried in the oil, the oil will probably contain enough peanut protein to cause a reaction.
- Any soups, stews, casseroles, or other blended dishes may contain peanut butter, ground peanuts, or peanut oil. Peanuts have shown up in dishes from chili to manicotti. Always ask about ingredients before ordering any dish.
- Beware the bread basket: we have encountered muffins made with peanut flour and pats of butter with ground peanuts blended in.
- Some imported tomato sauces and pastas contain peanut oil.
- Peanut oil is used in numerous pizza recipes.
- Certain cuisines—Chinese, Japanese, Thai, and African in

particular—rely so heavily on peanuts that cross-contamination is inevitable. Avoid these restaurants.

• Desserts are problematic. Any baked dessert may contain peanuts or enough peanut traces to cause a reaction. Best bets are ice cream—provided your server can tell you the ingredients—and fresh fruit. Many parents choose to bring their own special dessert.

Miscellaneous:

• Many foods for small animals such as guinea pigs and hamsters contain peanuts.

• Peanuts and peanut butter are very appealing to wildlife, so they are often found in bird food and seed dispensers.

• Peanut butter is the lure of choice for mice. If you need to call in exterminators, be sure to tell them to carefully hide all mousetraps.

• Lotions and creams may be made with peanut oil. Read every label carefully.

TREE NUTS

At the deli counter:

• Tree nuts may be added to salads. If any one salad in the deli case has tree nuts, there is a good chance for cross-contamination to occur with the other salads.

• Pasta salad may be made with pesto, which usually has piñon nuts as an ingredient and often walnuts as well. Always ask.

At ice cream and candy stores:

• Nuts or nut oils may be in any candy at all. If a nut-free candy is stored with candy containing nuts, the nut-free candy must be considered unsafe to eat. Only allow your child to eat wrapped candy with an ingredients label that you can read.

• Ice cream shops use the same scoops for all ice cream flavors, so cross-contamination is a given. If possible, order your child a soft-serve cone, after you have determined that no nuts are in the flavor and no nut flavor has been served from that machine for a few days at least.

In restaurants:

• Salads may have nuts tossed in or may be dressed with a nut oil.

• Slivered almonds may be tossed with vegetables or served on top of fish or chicken. If this is the case, simply removing the nuts does not make the food safe to eat.

• Ground nuts may be found in virtually any dish that calls for ground meat or chicken, from ravioli to spicy meatballs. Always ask.

• Breads frequently contain bits of nuts.

• If you notice a special fried entree that features nuts—pecan-crusted fried chicken, let's say—assume that the cooking oil has enough nut protein in it to cause a reaction, and do not allow your child to order fried food. Occasionally, french fries will be cooked in their own separate fryer. Ask if this is the case.

• It's safest to assume that baked desserts either contain nuts or have been cross-contaminated with nuts. Ice cream or pudding may be a good choice if your server can check on the ingredients. Fresh fruit with whipped cream (make sure the whipped cream isn't flavored with a nut extract!) may be another good choice.

At the grocery store:

• Many more cereals than you'd expect contain nuts, particularly those touted as *multigrain* or that have the word *healthy* in their name. Granola almost always contains nuts, as do granola bars.

• Many whole-grain breads contain nuts or carry a warning about possible cross-contamination.

• Cookies and crackers may contain ground nuts.

Miscellaneous:

• Pet food for small animals may have tree nuts.

• Personal care products such as shampoos, body oils, creams, and lotions may be made with nut oil.

WHEAT

Although all food-allergic children would do best to avoid processed foods whenever possible, those who are highly allergic to wheat benefit most of all. Although many processed foods do not contain wheat or wheat protein, the vast majority do. As always, the fewer ingredients there are in a food, the better.

At the deli counter:

• Many sandwich meats are made with cereal fillers or modified food starch, which frequently has a wheat component. (If the ingredient merely says "starch," you may safely assume that it's cornstarch.) Hydrolyzed vegetable protein or hydrolyzed plant protein frequently contains wheat. Read the ingredients on the meat to be sliced before allowing your child to eat it. If your child is anaphylactic to wheat, understand that there is a risk of cross-contamination if meats with cereals or modified food starch are sliced on the same equipment.

• Processed cheese may also have a wheat component. Exercise the same caution as above.

• Dressed salads may contain soy sauce, which contains wheat, or other wheat-derived substances such as wheat germ oil. Turkey salad may have been made from a prebasted bird, and most basting sauces have wheat in them. Fruit salads stand the risk of cross-contamination from their neighbors. You're best off avoiding premade salads.

At the grocery store:

• Do not assume that rice, corn, or oat cereals are wheat-free. Many such cereals are loaded with substantial amounts of wheat. Always read the label carefully.

• Be especially wary of sauces, gravies, and dressings, both savory and sweet, from tomato sauce to soy sauce to oyster sauce to chocolate sauce. You'll find at least some wheat protein in most of them.

• Along the same lines, avoid any foods that may have been marinated or prebasted.

• Most canned soups are another place for wheat to hide. Read the labels carefully.

• Many ice creams, sherbets, sorbets, and Italian ices are made with some form of wheat.

• You'll even discover wheat in most chewy candy—licorice, jelly beans, gumdrops, candy corn, and the like. Many brands of plain chocolate are safe, but it is a little-known fact that candy manufacturers often use flour on their production lines to keep the candy from sticking as it is processed. This is a perfectly safe and wholesome practice in general, but not for those with wheat allergies. To find out if this is the case with your family's chocolate of choice, contact the manufacturer directly. And of course, read all the labels.

• Many hot cocoa mixes are made with wheat starch.

• Although rice is a wheat-allergic child's best friend, most rice *mixes* will have some wheat ingredients in them too. If your child has a hankering for specialty rices, learn to whip up a quick and easy risotto. Your whole family will be the richer.

• Shredded cheeses and processed cheeses usually contain some form of wheat starch or wheat protein.

• Many brands of yogurt use modified food starch as an ingredient, which may indicate the presence of wheat protein. Stick to the brands that are simply cultured milk, sweetener, and safe flavorings.

• Frozen vegetables in sauce will probably have some form of wheat or wheat protein.

• Here's an unusual one: the glue used on many envelopes,

stamps, and stickers gets some of its sticky quality from wheat starch. Use the self-stick kind or a sponge.

At ice cream and candy stores:

• Although some brands of ice cream have many wheat-free flavors, if there is a fudge-brownie or cookies-and-cream variety you have to assume that the flavor your child wants has been cross-contaminated with a wandering ice cream scoop. Call the manufacturer to determine the ingredients of the soft-serve varieties, if any. And of course, the cone is a no-no.

• The only safe candy is a candy that's prewrapped, with the ingredients clearly marked. Individually wrapped chocolate bars, hard candies, and chewy candies may all be perfectly safe so long as you can read the ingredients.

In restaurants:

• Stick to plain grilled foods such as chicken, fish, steaks, and chops, *without sauce or marinade*. Depending on the severity of your child's allergy, a hamburger that arrives on a bun may have enough wheat protein on it even after the bun has been removed to cause a reaction. (And the hamburger itself may have bread crumbs in it—always ask.)

• Avoid fried foods. They will have been cooked in the same oil as breaded items.

• Desserts such as puddings and ice creams may contain food starch. Your child would do better with fresh berries and whipped cream, granita (available in Italian restaurants), sorbet (once the ingredients have been checked), or a nice dessert from home.

SOY

Any processed food picked at random off a grocery shelf stands a good chance of having some form of soy in the ingredients. Soy flour, hydrolyzed vegetable protein, and soy protein isolate are the most common forms. In general, soybean oil and soy lecithin are considered safe for soy-allergic children, but be sure to consult your allergist to make sure this is the case for *your* child.

At the deli counter:

• Many deli meats, franks, and sausages have soy additives. Always read the ingredients.

• Soy protein may be present in canned meats and fish, so avoid the deli salads.

• Bread, rolls, and English muffins may contain soy flour or soy protein. If you are ordering a sandwich for your child, make sure you know the ingredients of the bread.

At the grocery store:

• *Any and all processed foods may contain soy.* The most common offenders are canned soups, rice mixes, cereals, crackers, cookies, candy, breads, muffins, baking mixes, snack bars, meat or chicken coating mixes, dairy-case dough, and frozen desserts, but soy protein may be found in virtually any processed food. Get R.E.A.L.: Read Every and All Labels.

At ice cream and candy stores:

• Finer ice cream stores seldom use soy in their products, but you must always check. When in doubt, soft-serve may be your best bet, as the chances for cross-contamination are slimmest. Always ask to read the ingredients. Ice pops and other wrapped treats are even safer, as they have the ingredients printed on the package.

• Pure chocolate candies are generally not a problem, but always check the ingredients. Confections such as candy corn, jelly beans, gummy candies, and the like frequently contain soy.

In restaurants:

- Chinese and Japanese restaurants use so much soy sauce and other soy products in their cuisines that the best route is to simply avoid them.

- Soy sauce and teriyaki sauce are common ingredients in marinades, stuffed dishes (such as stuffed mushrooms), soups, stews, and salad dressings but may be used to enhance the flavor of any dish at all. Be sure to alert your server to your child's allergy when ordering any restaurant meal.

- Hamburger and hot dog buns are often made with at least a little soy flour.

- Margarine may include soy protein in the ingredients and may be used in restaurant cooking. Be sure to ask if this is the case.

- Breads in the bread basket may have been baked with soy flour.

- Although it would be the rare bakery that used soy flour or other soy products in cakes, cookies, and pies, the possibility does exist. The safest restaurant desserts are ice cream (if you can find out the ingredients), fruit ices, and fresh fruit with whipped cream.

13

FOOD ADDITIVES

A small percentage of children with food allergies will also react to common additives in foods such as food colorings, preservatives, and flavorings. These aren't true allergic reactions, per se—the immune system is not involved—but intolerances. The problem is, these additives are so omnipresent in our food supply that it can be hard to sort out precisely what is causing the reaction. Is your child wheezing after sucking on a yellow lollipop because the natural flavor included milk, egg, or peanut protein, or because of the yellow dye #5 (tartrazine)? Is that asthma flare-up due to an undeclared allergen in the granola bar or the sulfites in the bar's raisins?

While the actual number of children who are affected by additives *is* quite small, if your child is one of them numbers don't matter much at all. This chapter highlights some of the most commonly cited offenders. If you suspect that your child is sensitive to one or more of these substances, discuss your concerns with your health care professional. As always, avoidance is the path of least resistance, but some additives are easier to avoid than others.

Food dyes in particular show up in places you'd never expect. Many whole wheat products, for instance, while seeming the epitome of the unadulterated food, in fact contain yellow food dye to make them look more appealing. So before you cloak yourself in righteousness and banish all brightly colored sweets from your child's life, take a good look at the other foods he or she is eating. Chances are good that some wolves in sheep's clothing are also lurking in the pantry.

• *BHT.* This preservative, commonly added to breads and other baked goods, is safe and wholesome for almost everyone. Some children, however, seem to react to it.

• *MSG (monosodium glutamate).* The flavor enhancer long reviled for "Chinese Restaurant Syndrome," MSG is the sodium salt of glutamic acid, an amino acid found naturally in the human body and in all protein-containing foods. Most researchers think that the symptoms commonly attributed to an adverse reaction to MSG—most notably, an achy jaw—are probably triggered by some other substance in the food. Whatever the cause, reactions to MSG are generally mild and brief. Whenever MSG is added to a food, it is listed on the ingredients as monosodium glutamate.

• *Sulfites.* These preservatives, generally used to keep foods looking fresh or prevent the growth of microorganisms, have to be avoided by a small but significant number of children and adults. Fruits such as raisins, dried apricots, and figs frequently use sulfites to keep them wholesome. Other common sources of sulfites are soup and gravy mixes, jams, canned vegetables, fruit or vegetable preparations that might turn brown such as fruit salad or guacamole, juices, wines, shrimp, and maraschino cherries. Sulfite reactions can occur even when the exposure is extremely small, and are serious business: severe asthma can result. If you suspect that your child has a sulfite sensitivity, you must exercise the same caution and care that you would for a food allergy and never just assume that something is safe to eat without first reading the label or making inquiries.

14

PREVENTING ALLERGIES
IN YOUR *NEXT* CHILD

Now that you have one child with food allergies, the odds are tilted in favor of your next child having food allergies (or eczema or asthma or environmental allergies) too. But to paraphrase our feminist foremothers, biology is not necessarily destiny. There are some practical steps you can take to genuinely lessen the chances of your next child developing allergies. Of course, the key word here is *lessen*; a baby who comes into this world with a highly allergic immune system may very well develop allergies no matter what you do. But a baby with an average predisposition to developing allergies may not. Victory! Follow these guidelines, and you will ensure that your little one is growing up in the healthiest possible environment. Even if allergies do crop up down the road, you'll have the comfort of knowing that you did everything in your power to prevent them and may have at the very least blunted their impact.

For years, researchers have definitely demonstrated the positive effects of breast-feeding: the vast majority of babies who were breast-fed for at least six months have significantly less eczema, fewer respiratory infections, and a far lower occurrence of food and environmental allergies than their bottle-fed (or bottle-supplemented) peers. What's more, they are seldom overweight and may even have a slight edge in IQ scores as schoolchildren. Add to those benefits the warmth and intimacy of every feeding, and the case of breast-feeding is virtually ironclad.

However—there is always a *however* when it comes to allergies, isn't there?—mothers who are highly allergic themselves, whether to foods or environmental allergens, appear to pass the tendency on to their nursing infants. These babies develop more allergic reactions than babies of highly allergic mothers who are bottle-fed.

So what should you do if you know your baby is at high risk for developing allergies? The recommendations that follow outline the steps you should take. Every single one is important!

- If at all possible, make a 100 percent commitment to breast-feeding from the moment of birth on. That means not even an ounce of a milk- or soy-based formula in the hospital, which may set the stage for a future allergic reaction. If for any reason you are unable to nurse when your baby is hungry, and you have not yet expressed any breast milk for storage, it is safe to give your baby a hypoallergenic formula such as Nutramigen or Alimentum. Make sure that everyone who comes into contact with your baby in the hospital is aware of this stipulation. You might consider requesting that a small lettered sign reading "Hypoallergenic formula only" be taped to the isolette.

- Colostrum, the clear liquid produced by the breasts before your milk comes in, is an extremely useful substance for your baby. Along with bolsters for the immune system to fight infection, it contains a chemical called TGF-beta that actually boosts your baby's resistance to allergens. So be sure that your baby has a chance to nurse as soon as possible after birth and as frequently as possible in the first few days of life.

- While you are nursing, completely avoid major allergens such as dairy products, eggs, peanuts and tree nuts, fish and shellfish, and soy. Read every label! Some infants react to chocolate as well.

- If for any reason you are unable to breast-feed your baby, sticking to a hypoallergenic formula from the first feeding on is probably the wisest course. Check with your child's doctor.

• Delay the introduction of solid foods as long as possible. Wait until your baby is at least six months old. Then follow the advice most pediatricians give: to start with rice cereal and then proceed to other single-grain cereals (mixed with breast milk or water), then vegetables (yellow ones first), then fruits. Introduce each new food separately, and feed it consistently for three to four days before moving on to another one. Citrus fruits are generally not introduced until the baby is at least one year old and in your baby's case might be delayed even longer. Consult your older child's allergist as to when to introduce allergenic foods such as milk, eggs, wheat, and soy into your baby's diet, and do not introduce peanuts or tree nuts until your baby is at least three years of age.

• Protect your baby from developing environmental allergies by acting as if he or she already has them. *The single biggest risk factor for a child developing asthma or respiratory allergies is to live in a home with someone who smokes.* Do not allow anyone to smoke in your home. Do not carpet your baby's room or have any rug that cannot be run through your washer's hot cycle. Do not hang curtains or fabric wall-hangings. Wash your baby's bedding in hot water with unscented detergent. If you want to place one or two cuddly friends in the crib, be sure that they are washed every week in hot water, too. It goes without saying that a home free of furry or feathered pets is safer for a child with a tendency toward developing allergies, but if you already have a pet, make sure that it does not enter the baby's room and that you wash your hands well after playing with the pet. Ask friends and caregivers who have animals at home to do the same. (For more safeguards, see chapter 31, "Environmental Allergies.")

15

COMMUNICATING WITH YOUR CHILD'S HEALTH CARE PROVIDERS (AND YOUR HMO)

Your child's health care providers—that is, not just M.D.s, such as pediatricians and allergists, but also the physician's assistants and nurse practitioners who are playing an ever-larger role in health care—are the guardians of your child's health. So it makes sense to establish a cordial and reciprocal relationship with them from the very first visit. Far more than just good manners (which will be appreciated nonetheless!), it can even have an impact on the kind of care your child receives. If you are able to forge a warm, mutually respectful bond with your child's doctors, you will be listened to more closely and your "mother's intuition" will hold greater weight than in a less-attuned situation. You may get longer answers, more thorough explanations, and a more cheerful mood in the examining room. In short, a better encounter all around.

If this is your first visit with a particular doctor, or one that is bound to be stressful—scratch tests for a child who has been exhibiting pronounced allergic symptoms, for instance—you may want to bring a family member or trusted friend along with you. This third party can take notes, ask questions, and even watch your child for a brief period if you'd like some time alone with the doctor.

How Do You Find the Best Allergist for Your Child?

If you have a good relationship with your child's pediatrician, this should be the first person you ask when you're looking for an allergist. Chances are you will be referred to an allergist who specializes in children or who has a particularly good way with them. What makes a trusted pediatrician's recommendations particularly valuable is that he or she receives ongoing feedback from parents in the practice. If they aren't happy with the recommended allergist or find someone else they like even better, they generally let the pediatrician know.

If you're new in town or haven't been happy with your pediatrician's recommendations, you still have options. To find a board-certified allergist near you, visit these Web sites:

- The American Academy of Allergy,
  Asthma and Immunology
  www.aaaai.org

- American College of Asthma,
  Allergy and Immunology
  www.allergy.mcg.edu

Not surprisingly, the parents who are the most satisfied with their doctors are generally the ones who feel they have the most satisfying *communication* with their doctors. But communication can be a tricky thing. Some of the most highly regarded board-certified M.D.s can be sadly lacking in social skills. And similarly, some of the most loving, most concerned parents can appear pushy, ill-informed, or even laissez-faire when it comes to talking with their child's doctor. If we want the best for our children, somehow we've got to get together and make it work.

For better or for worse, the bulk of the responsibility lies with us. Drawing on my own and other parents' experiences of winters spent virtually camped out in the pediatrician's office, plus the input of a number of doctors, we came up with these simple guidelines:

1. *Start at the beginning.* The nurse or receptionist at the front desk is a hardworking employee with a name, a face, and a *memory*. It can seem like an effort to be polite and friendly when your child is unwell and you are anxious, but it is worth it. The quality of your child's care won't be affected by what she thinks of you, but what the other nurses think of your family might be. If you are brusque or otherwise unpleasant, she will no doubt pass that information on to her fellow employees. If you are consistently polite and friendly, she will likely pass that information on, too. If you don't believe me, just hang out in a doctor's office for a few hours and listen to what the people at the front desk chat about. When I worked in advertising, we used to call any gatekeeper to the executive suite—receptionist, executive secretary, or personal assistant—"White Fang," with all the respect and fear the term accorded.

2. *Look good.* It's an unavoidable fact of life that people treat you better when you're well-dressed and well-groomed. My mother-in-law dresses to the teeth whenever she has to bring her car in for servicing, and swears it works like a charm. So while no one expects the mother of two children under the age of three to be fully coiffed and outfitted in a stunning sportswear ensemble—especially when both children have been up wheezing all night—dressing a notch or two above your usual standards couldn't hurt. And if you find you are a little intimidated by doctors in general, it will help you level the playing field a bit. Of course, if you are one of those moms who always manages to look pulled together no matter what, you have probably sat next me or one of my friends in a doctor's waiting room one dismal February morning and wondered why we couldn't take a little more care with our wardrobe. Believe me, we were doing our best at the time.

3. *Come prepared with information.* Write it down on a notepad. Doctors work best when they have facts to deal with—that Betsy ran a fever of 101 for three days and broke out in a rash in a butterfly pattern on the fourth—rather than a story about Betsy feeling really hot for almost a week and then getting a rash toward the end of that time. It's not just a more efficient way of doing business; it's a way that doctors like and respect. When you're perceived as a parent who

accurately notes and reports her child's symptoms, the doctor will be more likely to respect your instincts and share both more time and information with you.

4. *Write down important questions.* How many times have you walked out of the doctor's office and realized within minutes that you forgot to ask the most important question you had? Don't let it happen again. Come prepared with a notepad and a pen to write down your doctor's answers. Don't go overboard—this is an appointment, not an interview—but be sure your major concerns have been addressed.

What if It's Just Not Working Out?

Like any relationship, the doctor-patient bond benefits from feelings of friendliness, mutuality, and reciprocity, and suffers from inattention, disrespect, and hostility. And sometimes, despite everyone's best efforts, personality types simply clash. If you have tried to establish an open line of communication with your child's doctor but believe that you are being belittled or are not being heard, it's best to listen to your heart and find someone else. You need to feel that your child's doctor is someone you can talk to, someone you can trust, and someone who will talk to and trust you as well.

Of course, there are interim steps along the way. If your child's doctor has an excellent reputation and comes with strong recommendations, yet you feel uncomfortable during that initial visit, it's probably worthwhile to give him or her the benefit of the doubt. Everyone, M.D.s included, has bad days now and then. If communication doesn't seem to be improving with subsequent visits, however, you might try gently expressing your dissatisfaction with "I" messages: "It's so important to me that you and I communicate well with each other. What can I do to make that happen?" You may be surprised at the positive response you receive from someone who had previously seemed cold, brusque, or harried.

If the relationship still doesn't improve, it's well worth the minor difficulty of finding another physician to feel that you and your child are among friends.

5. Once you've established a working relationship with your health care professional, you might find it helpful to *fax or e-mail information and questions to the doctor's office*, rather than waiting by the phone or playing phone tag to receive the doctor's or nurse's reply. Another benefit is that composing your message will force you to gather your information and frame your questions clearly. Of course, you give up a certain spontaneity, and your doctor may well have further questions before you can receive a satisfactory answer to your question. But for routine questions—should you increase the medication dose? which meds should you give when?—a fax or e-mail would be a viable way to go.

In short, the most informative, friendly, and useful doctor visits tend to be those that had the benefit of a little planning. It's a luxury we don't always have, but even a few notes and questions hastily jotted down—with answers duly noted—may represent a significant improvement.

DEALING WITH YOUR HMO

When everything is working smoothly—office visits and medications are covered; the right doctors are in the network; referrals are up-to-date—the HMO can feel like a real boon. But all it can take is one rejected claim to send your blood pressure soaring. Here are some guidelines from an insurance claims professional on how to get the most out of your plan.

1. *Pick the best plan from the outset.* If you or your spouse works for a mid- to large-size corporation, you probably have a choice of coverage plans within the HMO. Take the time to look over the options before you make your decision. For a child with health issues such as allergies and asthma, many insurance specialists favor the plans that are as close to "traditional" insurance as possible: for example, a plan that is fairly generous in terms of compensation for

out-of-network providers (including ambulance companies), and one that has a reasonable deductible for hospitalization, then covers 80 percent of the rest of the costs.

2. *Pay attention to the allergy clause in your contract.* Virtually all plans have one. The allergy clause will state how many tests (skin and RAST) the plan will cover each year, how often in a thirty-one-day period your child may visit the allergist (as opposed to the pediatrician), and how often you need to update your referral. If your child needs immunotherapy, there will be information about how many shots will be covered in a thirty-one-day period. (It is a source of some frustration that although a four-year-old may only need half the amount of serum as a fourteen-year-old, a shot is a shot as far as the HMOs are concerned.) The clause may also include details on how much medication (inhalers, antihistamines, steroids, etc.) will be covered in a given time period, and whether or not the plan covers equipment such a nebulizers.

In general, HMOs will cover as many skin and blood tests as your allergist deems it necessary to perform each year—but only *once* each year. You will probably encounter some resistance from your plan if an allergist believes the tests should be repeated after six months. To get the claim paid, you will at the very least need a firmly worded letter from the doctor and the help of your doctor's in-office insurance specialist.

3. *Make sure you understand asthma and pharmaceuticals coverage.* Asthma has been receiving better coverage from HMOs of late, but you may need to justify why your child is being seen by a specialist instead of a pediatrician. Once the reason is established, many HMOs are fairly generous in terms of how many visits per month will be covered.

Pharmaceuticals are another story. Most HMOs do cover prescription drugs, but that coverage is subject to contracts with pharmaceutical companies that may change at any time. You may have been routinely refilling your child's prescription for eight months, only to have the pharmacist tell you that the drug is no longer covered under your plan. Or you may need three inhalers for your child (one for home, one for the school nurse, and one for the after-school program your child attends), only to be told that your plan will cover only one inhaler in any given time period. Again, a strongly worded letter from your child's doctor and the diligence of the doctor's office staff can make all the difference. In cases of severe financial hardship coupled with recalcitrant HMOs, many doctor's offices will try to provide needy patients with free samples of medication when needed. If this is your situation—you truly have nothing you can trim from the family budget to accommodate the added burden of paying for your child's prescription medicine—by all means let your doctor know.

4. *Stay on top of your referrals.* Make a note of how often you need a referral. Most HMOs require that you update your child's referral to a specialist every six months. If the person in charge of insurance at your doctor's office is on the ball, ask him or her for help in getting your referral period extended to a year. It can be done.

5. *Don't be put off from going out-of-network.* Most people find that the most daunting challenge when dealing with HMOs is getting coverage for an out-of-network doctor. Here is where you must summon all of your powers of persuasion. Gather all the documentation you can as to why this particular specialist is the one to see, write a clear, forceful letter stating your case, and get a corroborating letter from your child's pediatrician. Enlist the help of your pediatrician's office staff. Then pray.

6. *Understand that you and your fellow employees have the power to change your plan if the benefits are not adequate.* Your company is a customer of the HMO. And like all other businesses, HMOs have to listen to their customers or risk losing them. If you know from experience that your child needs more coverage than the HMO provides, speak up. Better yet, ask around and see if there are others who are similarly discontented with the current plan. A common issue for allergy patients is how injections are handled. Some HMOs count receiving a once-a-week allergy shot the same as a doctor's visit. If you are only entitled to four doctor's visits a month, let's say, the injections alone will use up your allowance. But an injection is just an injection: ten seconds for the shot, twenty minutes in the

waiting room. You can make a solid case for why injections should not eat into your doctor-visit allowance. Make a list of how you would like to see your plan's coverage changed, with all the supporting reasons, then approach your benefits coordinator. Despite what you may think, there is some flexibility in every plan. A separate clause can be written for your company, but only if you actively work for it.

7. *Don't give up too easily.* Just received notification from your HMO that it won't cover that $75 for your daughter's visit to the E.R. on Christmas day? (Her asthma had flared from visiting Aunt Fran and her three cats, and no one was available at your doctor's office.) And now the hospital is sending you a scolding letter about your account being past due? Though you may feel (at times with justification) that you'd rather just write the check than deal with the hassle, if you have a solid case it may not be as hard as you think to get it resolved. Remember, insurance is a largely automated industry: just because a computer kicked back a claim doesn't mean it's a done deal. Call the 800 number on your insurance card and pitch your case. You may get a sympathetic ear. Just be sure to get the full name (or name and last initial) plus extension number of the person you speak to, and follow it up with a letter from your doctor's office stating why the treatment was needed. But if that fails, and you believe that you are truly being defrauded by your insurance company, the wisest course is to immediately . . .

8. *Contact your state insurance commissioner.* The office of the insurance commissioner acts as a Better Business Bureau of sorts for insurance claims in your state. You can find the phone number in your telephone book. When you call, you will be assigned a caseworker whose responsibility it is to do an independent internal evaluation of your case. From then on, the matter is basically out of your hands: the insurance company has to reply to the commissioner, and either justify to the commissioner's satisfaction why it denied the claim, or reconsider its position and pay the claim. Either way, time is of the essence in contacting the commissioner, particularly if the bill is very large or is causing you credit problems.

16

RECIPES

THE WHEAT-FREE CHALLENGE

Baking and cooking wheat-free are probably the biggest challenges in the food allergy pantheon. But as with all challenges, once you've negotiated a few crucial hurdles you can relax a bit and take the rest as it comes. For most families, that means getting an acceptable bread, a few kinds of baked goodies, and a pasta substitute in place.

If your child is allergic not only to wheat but to milk and egg products as well, the challenge is greater but by no means impossible. Remember: if the answer isn't where you are looking for it, it is where you are *not* looking for it. If your son turns up his nose at wheat-free pastas, perhaps your answer lies in cornmeal polenta cooked until firm, sliced thin, and layered like a lasagna. If wheat-free pizza crust is a dismal, cardboard-like affair, try my veggie-crust pizza. And if just the thought of baking wheat-free seems like too much to take on right now, beg the question with frozen desserts, chocolate delights, rice pudding, and other wheat-free staples.

WHEAT-FREE AND SWEET

Happily, wheat-free products are becoming easier and easier to find as more consumers eliminate wheat from their diets for all sorts of reasons. Most health food stores have a wide selection, and mail-order companies abound.

When it comes to prepared baked goods, however, nothing beats a good kosher bakery at Passover, the Jewish holiday celebrating the Exodus from Egypt. During Passover, which generally falls in April, observant Jews do not consume any grain products that have been leavened—that rose while baking—in commemoration of their ancestors fleeing Egypt before their bread had the chance to rise. A kosher bakery will have zealously cleaned out all its equipment in preparation for Passover, so there is a slim-to-none chance of any cross-contamination with wheat occurring.

While matzoh, a wheat-based flat bread, is traditionally eaten during Passover, baked items that need to rise usually rely on some combination of eggs and filling or potato flour instead. If your child can have milk and eggs, a true joy for the whole family awaits in the form of sinfully rich, velvety smooth flourless chocolate cake. In fact, if your freezer space allows, you may want to buy some extras to freeze in individual portions for birthday parties and other celebrations. Be sure to check with the bakery first to make sure that the cake is genuinely 100 percent flourless. Some specialty bakeries offer flourless chocolate cake all year long. You'll want to assure yourself that no obvious cross-contamination issues are present—mixing the flourless cake in the same, unwashed bowl as the other cakes, for example—but if you have found a safe source of flourless baked goods, you've found a gold mine.

Coconut macaroons, generally made with shredded coconut, sugar, eggs, potato flour, and possibly some almonds, are another chewy, delectable Passover treat that are available year-round, if not in the grocery stores and bakeries, then direct from the manufacturers.

Meringues, intensely sweet little cookies made from egg whites and sugar, are available in specialty shops and in many bakeries. Drizzle one or two with dark chocolate to satisfy even the most avid cookie monster.

And one of my personal favorites—chocolate-dipped fresh or dried fruit—is easy, versatile, and always delicious.

The best book I have read on living wheat- and gluten-free is Jax Peters Lowell's *Against the Grain* (1995, Henry Holt and Company). The author leaves no stone unturned in her quest for a tasty, wheat-free life, and offers plenty of recipes—many by acclaimed chefs who rose to her gluten-free challenge. You'll also find phone numbers and mail-order addresses of outside sources of wheat-free goodies sophisticated enough for adults but certain to please little ones as well. In turn, Ms. Lowell highly recommends Bette Hagman's *The Gluten-free Gourmet* series of books (Henry Holt and Company), calling them the home-baking bible for those living wheat- and/or gluten-free. Between these two books, you're covered.

CHOCOLATE DIXIES

I discovered this dessert quite by accident, when I was in a hurry and making a bigger mess than usual while icing chocolate cupcakes. The "Eureka" didn't hit me until a few weeks later, when I was talking to the mom of a wheat-allergic child about birthday treats.

These little molded cups are an easy take on what has always seemed to me to be a daunting process—molding chocolate to fit a form—and a quick, fun solution for wheat- or gluten-allergic kids when you don't have the time or energy to bake.

Makes about a dozen Chocolate Dixies.

2 cups semisweet chocolate bits	Allowed pudding, ice cream, or
2 tablespoons margarine or butter,	custard, plus candy garnish if
if allowed	desired

1. Fill a cupcake tin with paper or foil baking cups.

2. Melt together the chocolate bits and margarine or butter. In a micro-

wave, on high, this should take around 2 minutes. Stir until completely blended and smooth.

3. Put a heaping spoonful of chocolate in the center of each baking cup. Using a small spatula, spread the chocolate so that it completely coats the bottom and sides of the cup.

4. Put the whole cupcake tin in the refrigerator and chill for at least 30 minutes.

5. When the Chocolate Dixies feel firm, carefully peel off the paper baking cups. Fill your Chocolate Dixies with anything your child enjoys: pudding garnished with gummy candy, ice cream with allowed toppings, and creamy custard topped with a cherry are just some of your options. The fun part comes when you pick up your "cupcake" in your hands and eat the whole thing!

FRUITY OATMEAL BARS

My mother and I have been making these bars for years. They're quick, wholesome, and the perfect sweet to go with a cup of tea when those late-afternoon hungries hit. I've always loved them, but it wasn't until we had to go wheat-free for a few weeks that I truly appreciated them.

1 cup non-wheat flour (oat flour
  works well)
1 cup quick-cooking rolled oats
⅔ cup sugar
¼ teaspoon baking soda
½ cup (1 stick) margarine (or butter,
  if allowed)

Jar of your favorite fruit preserves
(apricot and raspberry work particularly well, but just about anything
goes)

1. Preheat oven to 350°.

2. Combine dry ingredients in a mixing bowl. Cut in margarine or butter until mixture resembles coarse crumbs.

3. Reserve half of the flour mixture. Press remaining mixture into an *ungreased* 9-by-9-by-2-inch baking pan.

4. Spread with jam and sprinkle with reserved flour mixture.

5. Bake for 30 to 35 minutes until golden brown. Cut into bars when cool.

CARAMEL OATMEAL BARS

These bars are about as simple as it gets—you don't even need a mixing bowl—but they are satisfyingly sweet and rich. If your child is a chocoholic, you can certainly stir in some allowed chocolate chips. Other add-ins that work are flaked coconut, snipped dates, and nuts, provided your child is not allergic to them.

1 cup brown sugar
½ cup butter or allowed margarine
1 teaspoon baking powder
2 cups quick-cooking oatmeal, uncooked

½ cup chocolate chips (optional)
½ cup flaked coconut (optional)
½ cup snipped dates (optional)
½ cup nuts (optional)

1. Preheat oven to 350°. Grease an 8-by-8-inch baking pan.

2. In a large skillet over very low heat, melt together the butter and the sugar, stirring constantly until the butter is completely melted and the mixture is a smooth consistency.

3. Remove from heat and add baking powder and oatmeal. Stir well. If you are adding any of the optional ingredients, stir them in as well.

4. Pour into the prepared baking pan and bake for 25 minutes or until the edges are brown. Cool on a wire rack. Let cool *completely* before cutting into bars.

RICE KRISPIES TREATS

These are the same old-fashioned favorites that were the hit of the PTA bake sale every year.

¼ cup allowed margarine
1 package regular-size milk-free, egg-free marshmallows

6 cups Kellogg's Rice Krispies Cereal

1. Grease an 11-by-17-inch baking dish.

2. Melt the margarine in a large pot over low heat.

3. Add marshmallows and stir until completely melted.

4. Remove from the heat and add Rice Krispies. Stir until the mixture is well-coated.

5. Pour into baking dish and flatten with a spoon. Let cool before cutting into bars.

Wheat-free at the Dinner Table

Considering all the delicious potato and rice dishes out there, it's not hard to make dining wheat-free a simple, easy pleasure. But it isn't without its challenges, either. A child who had already grown to love pasta and bread before a wheat allergy was diagnosed may sorely miss the spaghetti, rolls, breaded dishes, and pizza that were once a happy part of life. And because none of us relish the prospect of cooking separate meals every night, you probably want to prepare dishes your wheat-allergic child can enjoy with the rest of the family whenever possible.

Cooking wheat-free basically boils down to two categories: making substitutions, and going in a whole new direction. Some substitutions are surprisingly easy to make: quick-cooking oatmeal instead of bread crumbs in meat loaf and meatballs; or leftover rice instead of bread crumbs in vegetable quiches. Other substitutes are possible, but iffy: health food stores stock wheat-free breads and pastas, but not all children will eat them. Sometimes it's better not to fight it. Just follow a different direction: if the answer isn't where you're looking for it, it's where you're *not* looking for it.

OVEN-COOKED BARLEY PILAF

Not everyone loves barley, but I do. I like everything about it, from its tiny size to the hearty texture it lends to soups and stews. This barley pilaf can be made with rice if you prefer, but when you're eliminating wheat it's nice to have something from the grain family on the dinner table. This recipe is particularly good with roast chicken or with a dish that has a savory gravy, such as pot roast.

1½ cups boiling chicken broth
(check the label to make sure it's
wheat-free)
1 tablespoon vegetable oil

¾ cup quick-cooking barley
¼ cup *each*: sliced green onion,
chopped celery, chopped carrot

1. Preheat oven to 350°.
2. In a 1-quart casserole combine boiling broth and oil.
3. Stir in barley and chopped vegetables.
4. Cover and bake for 30 to 35 minutes or until liquid is absorbed.

CRUSTLESS QUICHE/WHEAT-FREE PIZZA CRUST

I used to make this dish with just spinach, artichoke hearts, and water chestnuts as the vegetables. My husband and I loved it, but our children wouldn't go near it. The addition of other vegetables (by all means add grated carrot, corn, or other vegetables your child enjoys) lessens the stigma of the spinach. If there is absolutely no way that your child will touch a dish with spinach in it, substitute chopped broccoli and handle with care—it won't hold together quite as well.

This versatile vegetable quiche forms its own crust as it bakes. You can serve it in fat squares or wedges, or spread the vegetable mixture thin in a round baking dish to create a "crust" for pizza. In the pizza version, it's best to allow the baked quiche to cool, then cut into wedges. Top each individual wedge with a little sauce and cheese and briefly run under the broiler (the microwave will make it soggy).

1 10-ounce package of frozen
spinach
3 cups assorted chopped vegetables:
mushrooms, onions, artichoke
hearts

2 large eggs
1 cup ricotta cheese (low-fat is OK)
1 cup shredded cheddar or Swiss
cheese (low-fat is OK)

1. Preheat oven to 400°.
2. Cook the spinach and squeeze out excess water.
3. Combine spinach with chopped vegetables, eggs, ricotta, and shredded cheese.

4. Spread mixture in ungreased round 8–9-inch or medium-size rectangular baking dish.

5. Bake for 30 to 40 minutes or until the quiche is browned around the edges and firm.

6. Allow to cool for at least 30 minutes before slicing.

POLENTA LASAGNA

Although polenta has a markedly different texture than pasta, this lasagna variation does still manage to satisfy that "soul food" craving so many of us get for hearty Italian dishes. Served with a crisp salad or a platter of raw vegetables and dip, it's wheat-free dining that everyone can enjoy. If your family enjoys meat sauces, by all means add ground beef to the recipe.

Note that the polenta needs to be cooked and chilled overnight before you can start the recipe. Preparing polenta is easy as 1-2-3, but you've got to get it done the night before!

1 box of polenta, prepared according to package instructions and chilled overnight in a greased rectangular baking dish

1 26-ounce jar of your family's favorite tomato sauce

1 cup ricotta cheese (low-fat is OK)

1 egg

1 tablespoon Italian spices (prepared mix or blend of oregano, basil, and thyme)

3 cups shredded cheddar cheese

½ cup Parmesan cheese

½ pound ground beef (optional)

1. Preheat oven to 350°.

2. Carefully turn out the polenta onto a cutting board and cut into medium (½ inch to ¾ inch) slices.

3. If you're using ground beef, cook it and combine with tomato sauce.

4. Mix together ricotta, egg, Parmesan cheese, and spices.

5. Lightly grease or spray a 9-by-12-inch baking dish and lay down first layer of polenta slices.

6. Carefully spread with ricotta mixture.

7. Top with half of the tomato sauce and 1½ cups of the shredded cheese.

8. Lay down second layer of polenta slices.

9. Top with remaining tomato sauce and shredded cheese.

10. Bake uncovered about 50 minutes, until sauce is bubbly and cheese is melted and slightly browned. Remove from oven and let stand at least 15 minutes before slicing.

Wheat-free in the Morning

Although the typical American breakfast appears to be one long parade of wheat products—bagels, cereals, toast, muffins, and pancakes—eating wheat-free at breakfast isn't as hard as it seems. A wide variety of wheat-free cereals featuring corn, rice, or oats are available at every supermarket (read the ingredients carefully to make sure no wheat starch or flour is going along for the ride), and frozen wheat-free waffles are beginning to turn up as well, although you may still need to visit a health food store for these. What's more, most children enjoy eating "lunch" foods such as sliced ham or turkey, yogurt, and cheese at breakfast as well.

The recipes included here are particularly useful for making breakfasts everyone in the family will enjoy. Other nice, easy breakfasts for wheat-allergic children are:

- Eggs (any style) with a small bowl of oatmeal or fruit
- Fruit and yogurt or fruit and cottage cheese
- Baked potato topped with shredded cheese
- Bowl of soup (why not?!)
- Peanut butter spread on fruit slices

GRANOLA

It can be challenging to find a wheat-free cereal that really satisfies, especially if your child has to avoid soy, which frequently means avoiding corn, too, because of possible cross-contamination. If your child is allergic to nuts, you need to avoid prepackaged granolas completely. Oats have the benefit of being high in protein and really sticking to your child's ribs. This simple, wholesome granola recipe is absolutely delicious served with milk at breakfast, stirred into yogurt, or spooned on top of ice cream. On cold winter mornings, heat some up with milk in your microwave. (Milk-allergic children can substitute soy milk, rice milk, or calcium-fortified apple juice.)

Are you a cereal sneak? (I am. A few handfuls of whatever sweet cereal my children are currently eating is my favorite before-bed snack.) If so, double the recipe—it won't last long!

2 cups rolled oats	½ cup raisins
½ cup honey or maple syrup	½ cup dates (snipped) or other
⅓ cup allowed oil	dried fruits

1. Preheat oven to 300°.
2. Stir oats, honey or syrup, and oil in a bowl. Spread mixture evenly into a greased cookie sheet.
3. Bake for 30 to 35 minutes, stirring after 15 minutes.
4. Remove from oven and turn out into large rectangular baking dish. Stir in dried fruit. Let cool, break into clumps, and store in tightly sealed container.

BAKING EGG- AND MILK-FREE

If your child is allergic to eggs, milk, or both, finding cakes, cookies, and other baked goods that the whole family can enjoy is a definite challenge. Luckily for us, a few venerable recipes such as shortbread and Wacky Cake are easy and delicious with no tampering at all. And just as luckily, Rosemarie Emro—daughter of a baker and mother of an egg- and peanut-allergic daughter—has taken it upon herself to make life delicious for egg-allergic children everywhere. Her book, *Bakin' without Eggs*, features more than 190 egg-free recipes for everything from pancakes, cookies, cakes, and donuts to Heavenly Brownies and an unbelievably rich and delicious cheesecake (assuming your child can have milk). It is truly a treasure trove for the food-allergic family. Although the emphasis is on egg-free baking, many of the recipes are milk-free as well, and others can be easily adapted for a milk-free diet.

ORANGE OAT BREAD
From Rosemarie Emro's *Bakin' without Eggs*

A not-too-sweet cakelike bread that's wonderful for breakfast with a little jam, or as dessert with a little confectioners' sugar on top.
    Makes one loaf.

2 cups unbleached all-purpose flour	½ stick milk-free margarine, melted
1 cup quick rolled oats	½ cup frozen orange juice concen-
1 cup sugar	trate, thawed
2 teaspoons baking powder	2 tablespoons grated orange peel
1 teaspoon baking soda	¾ cup orange soda

1. Preheat oven to 350°. Lightly butter a 9-by-5-by-3-inch loaf pan.

2. In a large bowl with a wooden spoon, mix flour, oats, sugar, baking powder, baking soda, margarine, orange juice concentrate, orange peel, and orange soda. Stir quickly until dry ingredients are moistened.

3. Pour into prepared loaf pan. Bake for 35 to 45 minutes or until tooth-pick inserted in center comes out clean.

4. Cool on wire rack in pan for 10 minutes, then remove from pan and cool completely on wire rack.

Copyright © 1999 by Rosemarie Emro, from *Bakin' without Eggs* by Rosemarie Emro. Reprinted by permission of St. Martin's Press, LLC.

BETTY'S GINGERSNAP COOKIES
From Rosemarie Emro's *Bakin' without Eggs*

This recipe makes approximately 3 dozen cookie-cutter cookies with a wonderful old-fashioned taste. Note that the dough has to be chilled overnight. This is an easy recipe, but you can't just whip it up on a whim.

2¾ cups unbleached all-purpose flour	¾ cup firmly packed light brown sugar
1 tablespoon grated cinnamon	3 tablespoons water
1 teaspoon ground cloves	3 tablespoons light molasses (dark
1 teaspoon ground ginger	will do in a pinch)
1 teaspoon baking soda	1 teaspoon lemon extract

1. In a large bowl, mix flour, spices, baking soda, and sugar. With a wooden spoon, stir in margarine until combined. Add water, molasses, and lemon extract. Mix thoroughly.

2. Cover bowl with plastic wrap and chill overnight.

3. Preheat oven to 350°. Lightly grease 2 cookie sheets.

4. Using a rolling pin, roll out dough to ⅛-inch thickness and cut with your favorite cookie cutters. Repeat until all the dough is used up.

5. Place dough on prepared cookie sheets ½ inch apart. Bake for approximately 8 minutes. Cool in sheets on wire racks 2 minutes, then remove with spatula to wire racks to cool completely.

[To make these holiday-specific, use the appropriate cookie cutters (hearts for Valentine's Day, evergreens or gingerbread men for Christmas, etc.), then ice with colored frosting after baking.—M.B.]

GRANOLA BARS

Most parents of peanut- and nut-allergic children have a well-justified fear of commercially packaged granola bars. With all the nut varieties floating around, there just seems to be too great a margin of error. But not only do kids love granola bars, they are a relatively nutritious treat, perfect for snack time or dessert. These granola bars are rich with raisins and chocolate chips, but you can certainly omit the chocolate if you feel that your child's sugar quota is more than adequately fulfilled every day.

Makes 16 bars.

1 cup firmly packed brown sugar
⅓ cup granulated sugar
½ cup milk-free margarine, softened
2¼ tablespoons honey
1 teaspoon vanilla extract
1 cup unbleached all-purpose flour
1 teaspoon cornstarch

1 teaspoon ground cinnamon
1 teaspoon baking powder
1½ cups quick rolled oats
1 cup crisp rice cereal
1 cup *each*, raisins and milk-free
   chocolate chips
¼ cup wheat germ

1. Preheat oven to 350°. Lightly grease a 13-by-9-by-2-inch pan.

2. In a large bowl, with a handheld electric mixer set on medium speed, beat sugars and margarine until fluffy. Blend in honey and vanilla. Slowly add flour, cornstarch, cinnamon, and baking powder; beat at low speed. With a wooden spoon, fold in oats, rice cereal, raisins, chocolate chips, and wheat germ until well mixed. Place in prepared pan and bake for 20 minutes until golden brown.

3. Cool completely and cut into bars.

ROSE'S OWN EASY CARROT-SPICE CAKE
From Rosemarie Emro's *Bakin' without Eggs*

This moist and delicious cake has a wonderful little secret: it's sugar-free! (If you really must, you can add some sugar, but it doesn't need it.) A perfect guilt-free treat!

2 cups firmly packed shredded carrots
2½ cups unbleached all-purpose flour
½ cup sugar (truly optional)
1 tablespoon baking powder
1 teaspoon baking soda
½ cup applesauce
1 6-ounce can frozen apple juice concentrate, thawed
½ cup water
1 teaspoon vanilla extract
2 teaspoons ground cinnamon
½ cup flaked coconut (optional)
½ cup raisins (optional)

1. Preheat oven to 350°. Lightly grease a 12-cup Bundt pan.

2. Put shredded carrots in a large bowl and slowly stir in flour, sugar (if used), baking powder, baking soda, applesauce, apple juice concentrate, water, vanilla, cinnamon, and coconut (if used). Fold in the raisins (if used) until completely mixed. If the batter is too thick to get a spoon through, add a little more water.

3. Pour into prepared pan and bake for 40 to 50 minutes or until a toothpick inserted in the center comes out clean.

4. Cool in pan on rack for 15 minutes and turn out onto a serving plate.

[This cake is also very good if you replace the carrots with grated sweet potato, substitute orange juice concentrate for the apple juice, and add 1 extra teaspoon of baking powder. You will probably need to bake this variation a little longer, but it's worth the wait.—M.B.]

WACKY CAKE

This cake is so easy and quick to bake, so versatile, delicious, and low-fat, it deserves to be part of *every* family's repertoire. It freezes beautifully, so make two at a time. You never know when you'll need a quick, special dessert. (Our son's school keeps individually wrapped, carefully marked squares of Wacky Cake in the freezer for him. They're prefect for parties or when a mom drops by unexpectedly with donuts or other goodies.)

For cupcakes, line your muffin tin with baking cups and reduce baking time by 5 to 10 minutes. This recipe makes 10 to 12 cupcakes.

1½ cups flour	1 teaspoon vanilla extract
1 cup sugar	1 tablespoon vinegar (balsamic
½ teaspoon salt	works beautifully)
3 tablespoons cocoa*	5 tablespoons oil
1 teaspoon baking soda	1 cup cold water

*For a chocolate-free variation, omit the cocoa and add ½ teaspoon of ginger, ½ teaspoon of cinnamon, and ½ teaspoon of cloves for spice cake.

1. Preheat oven to 350°. Mix dry ingredients in a bowl.

2. Add vanilla, vinegar, oil, and water. Blend well and pour into ungreased 9-by-11-inch rectangular pan.

3. Bake for 25 to 30 minutes.

TOPPINGS:

Plain confectioners' sugar and fresh fruit such as strawberries or raspberries make a light, elegant topping if the cake will be eaten all at once, that day. Otherwise, the confectioners' sugar will melt, making the top of the cake soggy and unappealing.

For an especially easy icing, all you need are whatever chocolate chips your child is allowed. About 1½ cups of chips, run through the microwave on high power for a minute and then stirred until all the chips have melted, should do it. Then simply spread the melted chocolate on the cooled cake. If you like a thin, crunchy chocolate crust, put the cake in the refrigerator. If you prefer soft icing, leave it out. Either way, it's delicious.

For a white icing, gradually cream together 4 tablespoons of butter, if allowed, *or* milk-free, soy-free margarine, with 2 cups of confectioners' sugar. Blend the sugar in, ½ cup at a time. When just ½ cup of sugar is left, add 3 tablespoons of milk or milk substitute to the frosting and beat with a spoon. Add the rest of the sugar and beat until smooth. Add 1 teaspoon of vanilla and a pinch of salt. Mix together and spread on cooled cake.

OIL DOUGH FOR SWEET AND SAVORY PIES

Quick to make and virtually foolproof, this dough takes the angst out of pie baking. Use it for everything from apple, cherry, and blueberry pies to chicken pot pie and meat pies. The crust doesn't really brown, so you may want to sprinkle a little cinnamon-sugar (available premixed or mix it yourself half and half) on top of your sweet pies just for color.

Makes enough dough for a two-crust 8-inch or 9-inch pie.

2 cups flour
1¼ teaspoons salt

⅔ cup Wesson or Crisco Oil (these
  two brands work best)
3 tablespoons water

1. Preheat oven to 450°.
2. Put the flour and salt into a large mixing bowl and stir together.
3. Add the oil and stir until the mixture is moist. Then add the water and stir well.
4. Kneading lightly, make a big smooth dough ball. Divide into two portions: ⅔ of the dough and ⅓ of the dough. The larger portion will be your bottom crust. Make evenly shaped patties from each portion.
5. Lightly dampen your work surface with a sponge. Place a sheet of wax paper (measuring at least 1 foot by 2 feet) on top. Place the larger patty on the wax paper. Tear off another sheet of wax paper that is the same size and place on top of the patty. Now you can roll out the dough without it sticking to the rolling pin. Roll it out until you have a nice, even circle between ¼ inch and ½ inch thick.

6. Peel off the top layer of wax paper and, holding the bottom layer of wax paper by the edges, turn the rolled-out dough upside down over your pie plate. Gently peel off the wax paper and ease the dough into the plate.

7. Fill with fruit or meat mixture.

8. Repeat rolling-out process for the top layer of dough and place it on top, crimping edges together. Score the top with a fork to let steam escape.

9. Bake for 15 minutes, then turn the oven down to 350° and bake for another 20 to 30 minutes, depending on your recipe.

ZUCCHINI BREAD

This dense, sweet bread is rich enough for a dessert but also delightful for breakfast. The crust gets nice and crunchy, while the inside stays moist. And the best part is, you get two loaves for the work of one!

The recipe freezes well, so resist the temptation to gobble down both loaves at once, and put one aside for a hurried morning.

Makes two loaves.

3 cups flour
½ teaspoon baking powder
1 teaspoon salt
2 teaspoons cinnamon
1 teaspoon baking soda
2 cups grated zucchini

4½ tablespoons water, 4½ tablespoons oil, 1 tablespoon baking powder, mixed together
1 cup good-quality vegetable oil
1 tablespoon vanilla extract
2 cups sugar

1. Preheat oven to 350°.

2. Grease and flour two 9-by-5-inch loaf pans.

3. Sift or whisk together flour, baking powder, salt, cinnamon, and baking soda.

4. Add remaining ingredients and mix well.

5. Pour into loaf pans and bake for 1 hour or until toothpick inserted near center of loaves comes out clean.

BANANA BREAD

When you're baking without eggs, even the most adaptable recipes can get a bit heavy and sodden. I was happy with this bread's taste but disappointed with its texture until I used an electric mixer to combine the ingredients. You don't have to mix the batter for long—2 minutes at most—but it definitely makes a difference.

Also, make sure that your bananas are nice and ripe, but not too large. Too much banana actually works against you. This recipe is good for muffins too. For a fun addition, throw in a handful of allowed chocolate chips.

½ cup oil

1 cup sugar

3 tablespoons oil, 3 tablespoons water, plus 2 teaspoons baking powder, mixed together

2 bananas, mashed

2 cups flour

1 teaspoon baking soda

1. Preheat oven to 350°.
2. Grease and flour one 9-by-5-inch loaf pan.
3. Combine all ingredients in the order given.
4. Mix with an electric mixer for 2 minutes.
5. Pour into pan and bake 45 to 50 minutes or until done.

Copyright © by the Food Allergy Network. Reprinted by permission of the Food Allergy Network.

SHORTBREAD (VERSION 1)

This classic recipe, always a baker's friend, is a true gift to those of us baking milk- and egg-free. Shortbread is the little black dress of cookies: dressed up (with chocolate bits, chopped dried fruit, icing, or candy decoration) or dressed down (with a quick sprinkle of confectioners' sugar or nothing at all), plain or sweet, it is always just right.

The recipe that follows is as simple as it gets. Use it as a canvas for your creativity. It doesn't get much easier than this!

1¼ cups flour

3 tablespoons sugar (taste and adjust upward if you prefer a sweeter cookie)

½ cup allowed margarine, or butter if allowed (go with butter if you can)

1. Preheat oven to 325°.

2. Combine flour and sugar. Cut in margarine or butter until mixture resembles coarse crumbs.

3. Form into a ball and knead until smooth.

4. Roll out on a very lightly floured board and cut into rounds, shapes, or strips.

5. Place 1 inch apart on ungreased cookie sheet.

6. Bake for 20 to 25 minutes or until bottoms just begin to brown.

Consider adding: ½ teaspoon each of cinnamon, allspice, nutmeg, and ginger for a spicy shortbread; 1 teaspoon grated orange or lemon peel for a fruity shortbread; 1 teaspoon of vanilla or lemon extract.

SHORTBREAD (VERSION 2)

This recipe is for a sweeter bar cookie. If you prefer your shortbread in wedges, just bake this recipe in two round pans and reduce the baking time by 5 to 10 minutes.

1 cup allowed margarine, softened*

1 cup brown sugar

1 teaspoon salt

2 teaspoons vanilla extract

2 cups flour

1 cup chocolate chips or 1 cup raisins or 1 cup snipped dates (optional add-ins)

2 teaspoons cinnamon-sugar (optional topping)

*If your child is permitted to have butter, by all means use it. This recipe is fine with margarine, but butter really does make a difference.

1. Preheat oven to 375°.

2. Cream together the margarine, sugar, salt, and vanilla extract until smooth.

3. Mix in the flour until well blended.

4. Add chocolate chips, raisins, snipped dates, or other add-in, if desired.

5. Spread into a greased 9-by-11-inch baking pan, sprinkle with cinnamon-sugar if desired, and bake for about 30 minutes. Shortbread doesn't really brown. You can tell it's done when the sides are just beginning to brown but the center is a mellow golden color.

6. While the shortbread is still hot, cut it into bars or into cookie-cutter shapes. Allow to cool in the pan before removing.

WORLD'S BEST CHOCOLATE CHIP COOKIES

Our family has become famous for these cookies. We bake them at least three times a week because they're a breeze to make and taste exactly like the Toll House cookies you may remember from childhood. The only thing to bear in mind is that these cookies don't keep in the cookie jar as well as cookies with eggs. (As soon as they've cooled, pack them in plastic containers or a storage-size plastic bag.) They do, however, freeze beautifully.

Makes about 2 dozen cookies.

1 stick margarine, or butter if allowed
½ cup sugar
1 teaspoon vanilla
½ teaspoon baking soda

1¼ cups flour
1 teaspoon baking powder, 1 tablespoon balsamic vinegar, and 1 tablespoon water, mixed together
1 cup allowed chocolate chips

1. Preheat oven to 375°.

2. Cream together margarine or butter with the sugar. Add vanilla, baking soda, flour, and baking powder mixture. Mix well with fork—the cookies do not come out as well if you use an electric or handheld mixer. Add chocolate chips and mix well.

3. Drop teaspoons of batter onto ungreased cookie sheet and bake for 11 to 13 minutes, until golden.

To make chocolate-chocolate chip cookies, add 2 tablespoons of unsweetened cocoa powder and increase sugar to ¾ cup.

BIRTHDAY CAKE

Here's a milk- and egg-free double-layer birthday cake that your child will happily share with classmates, family, and friends. No one will be able to tell the difference!

3 cups flour
1¾ cups sugar
1¼ cups water
½ cup allowed shortening
3 tablespoons water, 2 tablespoons

oil, 2 teaspoons baking powder,
  mixed together
2½ teaspoons baking powder
1 teaspoon salt
½ teaspoon vanilla extract

1. Preheat oven to 350°. Grease and flour two 8-inch round cake pans.
2. Combine all ingredients in a large bowl. Beat well with an electric mixer until batter is smooth—about 4 minutes.
3. Pour batter into prepared pans and bake for 40 to 45 minutes or until toothpick inserted in center comes out clean.
4. Cool in pans for 10 minutes. Finish cooling on wire racks. Frost when completely cooled. (See the frosting recipes that follow.)

Copyright © by the Food Allergy Network. Reprinted by permission of the Food Allergy Network.

FROSTINGS FOR DOUBLE-LAYER BIRTHDAY CAKE

Everyone knows that the frosting is what makes birthday cakes special. Luckily, it doesn't take much finessing to create a creamy, delicious frosting that milk- and egg-allergic children (and their families) can enjoy.

Cocoa Frosting

½ cup allowed margarine, softened
½ cup Hershey's unsweetened cocoa
  powder
2⅔ cups unsifted confectioners'
  sugar

¼ cup water
1 teaspoon vanilla extract

1. Beat margarine at medium speed in large mixer bowl until softened, about 1 minute.

2. Add remaining ingredients. Beat on low speed until ingredients are moistened, then on medium speed until creamy.

Creamy Vanilla Frosting

1½ cups allowed margarine, softened

4 cups confectioners' sugar

2 tablespoons water

1 teaspoon vanilla extract

1. Beat margarine at medium speed with an electric mixer until soft and creamy.

2. Gradually add sugar. Beat until light and fluffy.

3. Add water and vanilla extract. Beat until frosting reaches spreading consistency.

Copyright © by the Food Allergy Network. Reprinted by permission of the Food Allergy Network.

APPLESAUCE CAKE

This is a variation on a classic recipe that I have seen printed everywhere from the sidebar on catalogs to women's magazines. The spices vary from one version to the next, and some cakes call for the addition of raisins, chopped nuts, or both. Through a little trial and error, I've come to this formulation; but feel free to experiment—the cake is very forgiving. Interestingly, no matter where I've seen a variation of this recipe printed, no mention is ever made of the fact that the cake is milk- and egg-free. The recipe stands on its own merits.

2 cups flour

½ teaspoon salt

1 teaspoon cinnamon

½ teaspoon ginger

½ teaspoon nutmeg

1 cup sugar

½ cup allowed margarine

2 teaspoons baking soda

1¼ cups applesauce

1. Preheat oven to 350°.

2. Whisk together flour, salt, and spices in a large bowl.

3. Cream together the margarine and sugar and beat with an electric mixer on medium speed for 3 minutes until soft and blended.

4. Combine the baking soda and applesauce. Fold into the margarine-and-sugar mixture. Gradually stir in the dry ingredients until smooth.

5. Pour batter into a greased and floured 9-by-11-inch pan and bake for 45 minutes or until a toothpick inserted in the center comes out clean.

1-2-3 SANDWICH COOKIES

These easy, light cookies can be filled with your choice of jam, frosting, or simply melted chocolate. They can be mixed up in a jiffy; the only slightly time-consuming part is rolling and cutting out the dough. I like to use small heart-shape cookie cutters for this recipe, but any shape will work. If you want a bakery-like cookie, sprinkle the finished products with confectioners' sugar. Personally, I think they're grand just the way they are.

2¼ cups flour
¾ cup sugar
2 sticks allowed margarine
2 teaspoons vanilla

Jam or melted chocolate for
  spreading
1 teaspoon to 1 tablespoon water,
  as needed

1. Preheat oven to 325°.

2. Mix together flour and sugar in a large bowl.

3. Soften margarine and add to flour-and-sugar mixture. Add vanilla. Your final product should be a ball of dough. If the dough is too crumbly to make a ball, add a little water at a time until it reaches the proper consistency.

4. Dampen your work surface with a sponge and lay out a 2-foot-long sheet of wax paper on top. This is where you are going to roll out your dough. Pat your dough ball down to a flattened round and lay another sheet of wax paper on top. This will keep the rolling pin from sticking to the dough without adding unnecessary flour. Roll out the dough to ¼-inch thick and cut it in the shapes you choose.

5. Carefully place cookies on ungreased cookie sheets and bake for 10 to 12 minutes. The cookies should be a little soft and light-colored on top but slightly browned on the bottoms.

6. Cool thoroughly before filling.

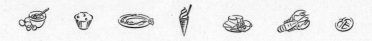

PART II

Coping

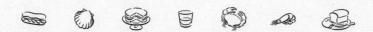

17

HELP AND HOPE: TWO ORGANIZATIONS THAT ARE MAKING A DIFFERENCE

THE FOOD ALLERGY NETWORK

It is no exaggeration to say that the Food Allergy Network (FAN) saved our lives.

Four years ago, when I walked out of Dr. Scott's office with a laundry list of foods Lucas had to absolutely avoid—milk, eggs, peanuts, tree nuts, corn, soy, tomatoes, green beans, and, for a brief period, wheat—I had no idea what I was going to feed him or how I was going to be able to keep him safe. I'd never read an ingredients list in my life—just blithely tossed items helter-skelter into my shopping cart. We were the only family I knew who had to deal with these issues. I didn't just feel overwhelmed; I felt utterly alone.

But Dr. Scott had pressed the FAN pamphlet into my hand as I left, and made me promise to call and join the organization as soon as I got home. So, numb and compliant, I did. I ordered almost everything FAN had to offer. (Details on how you can order from FAN are provided at the end of this section.) Within a week, my order arrived. And suddenly, everything seemed manageable. Here was an article about administering epinephrine. Here was a recipe for milk-free, egg-free, soy-free chocolate chip cookies and another one for chocolate cake. Here was a pamphlet that would help me explain food allergy issues and safeguards to the staff at Lucas's nursery school.

I was still a bit overwhelmed. But I was most definitely not alone anymore.

FAN was founded in 1991 by Anne Munoz-Furlong, whose daughter was allergic to milk and eggs. Frustrated by the lack of accurate information available on food allergies and by the prevailing attitude that food allergies don't need to be taken seriously, Anne saw the need for an organization that would act both as a central clearinghouse of medically sound, practical information and as a forum for all families dealing with food-allergy-related issues. FAN is now the largest organization in the world dedicated to food allergy and anaphylaxis.

FAN is a nonprofit organization with 22,000 members worldwide, including families, dieticians, nurses, physicians, school staff, government agency representatives, and people working in the food and pharmaceutical industries. Its stated goals are to help those with food allergies lead normal lives, manage their condition more successfully, and support research that develops a greater understanding of food allergy, its causes, and possible cures. Its focus is on children, because they are by far the largest group affected by food allergies. About 75 percent of FAN's members have a food-allergic child.

In the public arena, FAN works to build awareness of food allergy through media, education, publishing, advocacy, and research efforts. FAN is a founding member of the Food Allergy and Anaphylaxis Alliance (FAAA).

FAN is also an invaluable resource for the most up-to-date information on:

- Cooking healthy, delicious allergen-free recipes
- Shopping and reading food labels
- Planning trips and restaurant excursions
- Keeping your child safe at school, camp, and day care
- Helping your child feel "normal" at parties, holiday time, and while on vacation

- Handling health issues, from eczema to anaphylactic emergencies
- The latest medical research

Annual membership is currently $30. When you join FAN you will receive:

- The bimonthly *Food Allergy News*, a twelve-page newsletter packed with the latest on food allergy research, practical tips, dietary advice, recipes, and news.
- *Food Allergy News for Kids*, a four-page newsletter for children that includes stories and tips from youngsters who are dealing with the same issues as your child.
- Special allergy alerts, which contain urgent notices of mislabeled recalled food or pharmaceutical products, plus advance notice of ingredient changes from responsible food manufacturers.

All of FAN's publications are checked for scientific accuracy by its Medical Advisory Board, which consists of ten of the leading food allergy clinicians and researchers in the United States. FAN also provides a wide range of materials touching on every aspect of food allergy. For an up-to-the-minute list, visit FAN's Web site at http://www.foodallergy.org.

THE FOOD ALLERGY INITIATIVE AND
THE ELLIOT AND ROSLYN JAFFE INSTITUTE FOR FOOD ALLERGY

Established in 1998 by a group of parents who have children with severe food allergies, the Food Allergy Initiative (FAI) supports research to find a cure.

The Genomic Initiative, an FAI-developed study of the genetic makeup of food proteins that cause an allergic reaction, is the foundation upon which this groudbreaking research is based. The initiative for peanut was recently completed, and the future looks bright: all results indicate that an allergy shot against peanut-mediated reactions—a safe shot—is not only possible but quite probable. Dr. Hugh

A. Sampson of the Elliot and Roslyn Jaffe Institute for Food Allergy at Mount Sinai Medical Center (under whose guidance this book was written) has recently documented positive results in clinical trials. Under the leadership of Dr. Sampson, the institute has become the leading center in the United States for the diagnosis and treatment of food allergy. Once a cure for peanut allergy is found, that knowledge can be immediately transferred toward developing immunotherapy for other food allergies.

Although the focus is currently on safe shots, FAI is also following and supporting research involving other treatment strategies. In addition, FAI is working to see that centers similar to the Jaffe institute are established throughout the country, giving more food-allergic families access to the highest levels of treatment and care.

FAI also develops educational programs and public policy initiatives to increase awareness of the seriousness and severity of food allergies, so that no one will have to suffer a fatal food reaction again. In 1999, with New York senator Daniel Patrick Moynihan's support, the National Institutes of Health budget was increased by $200 million and has been directed to expand its research into food allergies. Efforts to pass legislation requiring that all emergency medical technicians be trained and authorized to administer epinephrine—the only treatment for an anaphylactic reaction—are also seeing results. At the time of this book's printing, Connecticut became the twelfth state to pass this lifesaving legislation.

Also in the works is an FAI pilot program to educate culinary students across the United States about food preparation to avoid cross-contamination with allergenic foods.

FAI wholeheartedly supports the Food Allergy Network in its efforts to increase the distribution of educational materials to schools, day care centers, and camps, and to produce additional videos related to food allergies. Anne Munoz-Furlong is a frequent guest and speaker at FAI events.

To find out more about the Food Allergy Initiative, either write to the organization at 625 Madison Avenue, New York, NY 10022, or visit its Web site: safefood@fai-web.com.

18

ORGANIZING YOUR KITCHEN

As my husband will be the first to tell you, I am not an organized person by nature. But unless you've known me for over five years, that might come as a surprise. In fact it still surprises *me* when friends will say, "Oh, but you're always so organized." I guess I am, but that's only because I have to be. That overstocked jumble that used to be my pantry is now as disciplined and tidy as a battalion of marines. For the kind of person that I am—all too often doing and thinking at least two or three things at once—to do anything else would be playing fast and loose with disaster.

Your approach to organizing your kitchen will depend on the kinds and severity of your child's food allergies and whether or not your family feels comfortable with keeping allergenic foods in the house. Of course if your child is allergic to staples like milk, eggs, or wheat, chances are you will continue to have those foods in your household. You'll just have to work around them. It seems to me that every family approaches the cupboards-pantry-fridge issue in its own way, within certain basic parameters.

But before you even begin to go through your cabinets and

refrigerator, you need to answer one basic question: how strict are you going to be?

Some people whose children are dairy and/or egg allergic will keep a few of those items in a special place in the refrigerator but will not stock any other items—including lunch meats, puddings, sauces, pastas, crackers, cookies, snack foods, or cereals—that contain milk or egg ingredients. They believe that the quart of milk, package of cheese, and dozen eggs are a necessary evil, but that their child should be able to safely eat anything else in the house.

Other families, confronted with the same restrictions, go in virtually the reverse direction: their household and household foods remain the same. But a special shelf in the fridge and a special shelf in the pantry are reserved for the allergic child's "safe" foods, which are marked in a certain way.

Still other families strive, for the most part, to stock their refrigerators and kitchen cabinets with foods that are safe for everyone to eat. But certain treats that would simply be too heartbreaking for other family members to give up—individually wrapped packages of cheese and crackers, say, or milk chocolate Hershey's Kisses—are bought sparingly and placed in a marked, sealed container high out of reach.

Our family used a combination of these approaches. When Lucas was allergic to many foods, including peanuts, milk, eggs, corn, and soy, I always had the same special food set aside and marked just for him. In fact, he ate the same brands of cereals, crackers, hot dogs, pretzels, and the like, for two solid years. (Luckily, that's playing right into most young children's preferred way of eating, anyway.) The beauty of that approach was that very quickly it became a no-brainer: all of us knew what constituted "Lukie food" and wouldn't dream of giving him anything different. (You do have to read the labels on each and every food item you purchase, however. Ingredients can and do change at any time, and in different parts of the country.)

The one thing I would not keep in my house under any circumstance was a product containing peanuts. Lucas was highly allergic to the other foods, but he was anaphylactic to peanuts. And having experienced the effects of peanut ingestion once, I was absolutely clear that it was not going to happen again—at least where I had control over it.

Now, in the past two years, I've slightly modified my plan. My older son adores certain snacks and candies that carry the warning "may contain peanut traces," and I want him to be able to have them. I keep a limited quantity of these, to pack into his lunch box, on the very high top shelf of our pantry. He does not eat them at home. (I am still not so brazen as to allow foods containing actual peanuts, and yes, I still dearly miss peanut butter.) The boxes I store these forbidden goodies in are boldly labeled *NFL* (Not For Lucas). I also point them out to Lucas and tell him that these products are not safe for him to eat. On the very rare occasions when my older son has a peanut treat in the house—a peanut butter cup in a party bag, let's say—I ask him to eat the treat in his room and to wash his hands afterward. If the bag is loaded with peanut items, I ask him to select the two or three items he wants the most. He eats those right away, and the rest get thrown straight in the trash.

It's all a balancing act: how much freedom you can give your peanut-loving people versus the safety of your peanut-allergic people. No one wants to feel that they're punishing other family members, but there are limits and restrictions in *any* group situation, regardless of whether food allergies are part of the mix.

One nice addition to our peanut-free pantry has been soy butter, which can be found in most health food stores. The taste and texture are very similar to peanut butter, and both my older son and my husband swear by it with raspberry jam on whole wheat bread. Soy butter is also much lower in fat and very high in protein. I can rest assured that if there's a tiny dab of soy butter on the counter, and Lucas comes into contact with it, he's not in any real danger. However, although Lucas is no longer allergic to soy, I would not serve soy butter to him or any other peanut-allergic child.

The number one argument against soy butter, or any other nut butter for that matter, is the opportunity for cross-contamination. Although the labels often make a big deal of saying that the product is peanut-free, I know that most nut butters are processed on shared equipment. You show me a processing plant that can get every last bit of peanut butter out of a machine, and I'll show you Santa's workshop, complete with Q-tip-wielding elves.

The second argument is that soy butter is just too much like peanut butter for comfort. It certainly looks just like it, and it even sort of smells like it. If your peanut-allergic child is used to eating soy butter, how is he or she going to tell the difference when confronted with two sandwiches, one safe, the other not? A child who is allergic to peanuts *should* hear alarm bells when a peanut butter–like substance is in the immediate vicinity, with no thought in mind that this might be a safe food. Being a person who's not too big on taking chances, I believe that our children should avoid the brown, sticky stuff at all costs, whether it's in a sandwich, on a tabletop, or spread in a celery stick and topped with raisins.

GETTING DOWN TO BUSINESS

The time has come to confront your kitchen. This can be a fairly lengthy, painstaking process or a quick, brutal one. It's up to you. I tend to favor the slash-and-burn method—toss most of it and start from scratch—but it doesn't matter how you go about the process. Your only goal is to create an environment that keeps your child safe.

Do your research:

1. Keep on hand for ready reference a printed list of ingredients that may indicate the presence of an allergen. (See the chapters in this book on specific food allergies.)

2. If you haven't done so already, read chapter 12, "Hidden Allergens." You may very well have some items in your kitchen that do not list your child's allergy trigger in the contents, but which pose a risk nonetheless. If you have already read chapter 12, reread it, taking note of the various foods listed.

Prepare to work:

3. Select a time to do the Big Clean-Out, preferably when the kids are out of the house or tucked into bed. Depending on how big your household is and how well stocked you keep your kitchen, you may need two to four hours to get the job done.

4. Clear a table or large countertop to be your staging area. You will be completely cleaning out one shelf at a time, moving all of the food from the refrigerator and cupboards to this one spot.

5. Gather some felt-tip pens or stickers and plastic containers. You will be using these to label and/or separate foods.

Get it done:

6. Choose your starting point, whether it's the refrigerator or the cabinets. In a systematic fashion, clear one shelf at a time onto your staging area. Examine each food item in turn, reading the ingredients for *all* processed foods. As the "Hidden Allergens" chapter points out, you can't take anything for granted: that bottle of vanilla extract most likely contains some corn syrup, and the baking powder probably includes cornstarch—both no-no's for corn-allergic children. The candy corn and cheese crackers may contain peanut traces. The soy sauce has wheat in it. The crackers may contain whey. Et cetera.

7. The foods that are safe go right back on the shelves. Depending on the system you've decided to use, either throw away all opened packages of unsafe or questionable foods, or clearly mark them as unsafe for your child to eat and store them together. Marking foods clearly is extremely important, since chances are good that over the course of a year there will be at least one or two occasions when someone other than you will be feeding your child. A good rule of thumb is to ask yourself: would a baby-sitter or neighbor be able to immediately tell that my child shouldn't eat this?

8. We filled a basket with *unopened* cookies, crackers, tins of nuts, and peanut butter and donated them to our local food pantry, but not everyone chooses to be so rigorous. If you decide to keep foods that pose a life-threatening danger to your child, put those items in a well-sealed, well-marked container and store in a hard-to-reach part of your kitchen.

9. When organizing a refrigerator, many families of dairy- and egg-allergic children find that it helps to keep all the unsafe items—lunch meat to cookie dough—in one compartment, which they mark. You would probably also want to mark the individual packages, just

in case someone forgets to put something back in the right place. The children quickly learn that they can help themselves to anything in the refrigerator *except* the items in that particular drawer. It also increases mindfulness for the parents: if you are opening a special drawer for the cheese, you get an extra jolt of awareness that your child can't have it.

10. Be wary of cross-contamination. If you store different kinds of cookies, cereals, or snack foods together in one big canister, *none* of the items are safe for your child to eat if *one* of them isn't. Chocolate sandwich cookies stored in the same bin as pecan shortbread might as well be pecan-studded themselves. By the same token, if you are emptying a canister of unsafe food, be sure to carefully wash it out before storing safe food in it.

Jars of jam and jelly are notorious for harboring unwelcome guests. If you've ever dipped a knife into the jam after dipping it into the peanut butter or spreading butter on toast, you know what I'm talking about. Most families, especially those with young children, have more than jam in their jam. If that poses a problem for your child, throw it out.

11. Now it's list-making time. You may find that after reading every ingredients label, you don't have a single box of cereal, crackers, or cookies that your child can safely eat. This is particularly true for kids who can't eat wheat, soy, or corn, which seem to show up in one form or another in almost everything. Not a problem. Really. Write down what you need to buy, then plan on making a trip to the grocery store, and possibly one to the health food store as well, if you have a nice large one near you. While it's easy to find national brands of food staples that are nut-, milk-, and egg-free (I'd rather not give you brand names because ingredients may change at any time), a good health food store is a veritable treasure trove for everything else, from canned soups to margarine to pancake mix. (I used to joke that when the manager at our local health food store saw me coming, he knew he'd make payroll that week.)

After you have gone through every last shelf in your kitchen cabinets, refrigerator, and freezer, reorganized your foods, and made your shopping list, there still might be one more step you need to take to completely protect your child. Children who are severely allergic to commonly used cooking ingredients such as milk and eggs may be better off having a few pans and cooking utensils plainly marked and set aside for their use alone. That way, you won't find yourself always minutely inspecting the frying pan and spatula that just came out of the dishwasher but might still have a tiny amount of egg on them, or constantly repeating some other similar behavior. The whole point of being well organized is to make things easy on yourself, so do whatever you have to do. In the long run, it will save you time and aggravation. And it will help keep your child that much safer.

19

LIVING GRACEFULLY IN THE REAL WORLD

While it's certainly true that a journey of 1,000 miles begins with a single step, we parents of food-allergic children need to remember that *our* first step must happen in our minds, long before anyone's foot hits the road. Because if that first step is off-balance, the whole journey may very well feel that way too.

What I'm talking about here is attitude—toward ourselves as capable parents, toward our children as precious gifts, and toward the world at large as willing and able to help us, if we help them too.

It's useful to keep in mind that although food allergies are a constant, demanding presence in *our* lives, a good many well-meaning, intelligent people we meet will have little knowledge or experience in dealing with a food-allergic child. It can be frustrating and even a little nerve-racking depending on the situation, but it really, truly does not mean that they will not be amenable to helping us, provided we give them the tools. Let's face it: we all have our own radar screen that can only process a limited field of information at a time. To keep the equipment in working order, what we don't need to know simply doesn't show up on the screen.

Each one of us will have many opportunities to be ambassadors, if you will, for all food-allergic children. Like all diplomatic matters, your relationship with the world at large thrives on small but significant courtesies: calling restaurants at off-peak hours to speak about food preparation with the manager or chef; perhaps even making a conscious effort to patronize restaurants at off-peak times, whenever possible, so that any extra preparations on your child's behalf won't tax an already maxed-out staff; approaching new people in the spirit of friendly cooperation; and dropping a brief note in the mail to personally thank restaurant or hotel personnel who have extended themselves for your family. At some time or another, all of us will be the beneficiaries of families who have graciously paved the way, whether by educating the owner of an ice cream shop on how to avoid cross-contamination, preparing a teacher or camp counselor for the responsibilities of caring for a food-allergic child, or by forming a bond with a waitress at a local restaurant. My friend Ellyn has been our family's guardian angel in that respect: her son is one year older than Lucas, and we've been on the receiving end of all the good work she's done with the school system and our local YMCA. Imagine my relief when on the first day of camp Lucas's counselor cheerfully informed me that he knew exactly how to take care of peanut-allergic kids and promptly rattled off every possible precaution—he'd had Ellyn's son the year before.

In turn, each of us has the chance to make life a lot easier for those who come after, by making sure that every one of our interactions is as friendly and positive as possible. It's human nature: if the first experience a person has with a food-allergic family is good, that person will be more likely to react positively the next time the issue arises.

Of course, not everyone will be as willing to make allowances for our children as we'd like. My family has had experiences in restaurants ranging from the divine (a chef who made special french fries in fresh oil for Lucas because the kind his restaurant served had an egg-batter coating) to the distressing (a waitress at an Orlando pizza parlor who launched into a diatribe about how people with serious food allergies were taking their lives in their hands by even stepping foot into a restaurant). A certain degree of latitude has to be factored in for time and place: the wonderful chef was serving us at 6 P.M. on Sunday, not 8 P.M. on Saturday; and the hysterical waitress looked to be handling about twice the usual limit of tables. Still and all, the chef was probably a helpful sort from the get-go, while the waitress probably overreacted to *any* special request.

It helps to fine-tune or perhaps even modify our perceptions of what is "owed" us in certain situations. Although you may feel in your heart of hearts that the world should make every effort to accommodate your child, as a purely practical matter it's not going to happen and you're going to feel put out and resentful. Better to adjust your expectations downward to pure safety concerns—that the people in charge of preparing food will be honest about their ingredients and what they can and cannot do for your child—and be pleasantly surprised if more than that materializes. Not infrequently it will, and you'll be in the happy situation of both receiving an act of generosity (theirs) and performing one (your wholehearted gratitude and personal thanks).

Occasionally, employees of a restaurant, bakery, or other purveyor will tell you that the establishment won't guarantee *anything* it sells to be free of your child's forbidden foods. It doesn't really matter what the motivation is: fear of legal liability, small-mindedness, or just simple ignorance. Accept it as the truth. Be grateful that they told it to you straight, thank them cheerfully, and move on.

This does not mean to say that your child has no rights at all. Like all other restaurant patrons, kids with food allergies have the right to eat food that will not make them sick. If, despite all of your precautions, your child does have a reaction to a food that was certified safe by the restaurant staff, it's well worth your time to investigate the cause once the reaction has been controlled. I think it's best to assume that the restaurant meant well and that an honest mistake was made, but restaurants do need to know how serious for the child the consequences of mistakes can be. They need to be made aware of how cross-contamination occurs, and how even a speck of the wrong food can be a major issue. In other words, if there is an accident, there should also be some learning that follows. And in my personal experience, if you treat the other person as if you're both on the same team trying to achieve the same goal, then the odds are good that you will be.

Some parenting books talk about a "teachable moment," which can occur when your child's emotions are slightly heightened, whether he or she is *beginning* to feel anxious, frustrated, angry, balky or has just achieved a small victory.

One of the premises of the teachable moment is that when you help someone overcome a *challenge*, that person takes away far more than in other circumstances. Consider the following example: Your daughter is not particularly good at spelling, and this week's words are exceptionally difficult. She's having a hard time getting them right, and you can see by the way she's starting to kick her shoe on the leg of her chair that frustration is starting to get the better of her. Now, when her mood could still go either way, is your moment.

You approach her with a smile. You hand her a glass of juice and tell her how proud you are that she is really trying and sticking with it. Then you offer her an option: perhaps you've come up with a silly rhyme that will help her remember one of the tricky words—can she come up with another? She does, and she's delighted. Instead of scolding her or watching her get more and more frustrated until she melts down, you've lightened the mood and taught her a new skill— a skill she can call upon again and again.

The same sort of situation occurs every time food-allergic families need to enlist the help of someone who is new to the whole business. As you express your request, you can assume that the new person is starting to feel some heightened emotion, whether it's anxiety, impatience, confusion, pride in being responsible, or irritation at feeling overburdened.

Remember that not only are you asking, you are *teaching*. You don't need to give a wealth of background information, but you should always be very pleasant, matter-of-fact, and clear about what you need and why you need it. Give the new person a full acknowledgment that he or she is going above and beyond the call of duty, and freely express your gratitude when you receive what you've requested. (A handsome tip to a waiter who has gone the extra distance for your family is certainly in order.) Each time you successfully negotiate a situation like this, you gain confidence in your ability to move freely in the world, and someone new has learned how to help a food-allergic kid.

Just as your friendly, can-do attitude paves the way for your child's safety, it also helps your child learn how to deal with the outside world. If our children see us approaching new people with warm courtesy, that will be their inclination as well.

20

HOLIDAYS AND SPECIAL OCCASIONS

Holidays are what childhood memories are made of, and food is an integral part of it all. When I was growing up, it seemed that I could taste the seasons as they circled round: toasted pumpkin seeds and candy corn were fall; hot cocoa and peppermint sticks were winter; asparagus (I loathed them; my mother loved them) were spring; orange ice pops and hot dogs were summer. We ate pizza on Friday nights, Chinese food on the Fourth of July (a tradition that began with my mother's Brooklyn childhood), and deli smorgasbords after funerals. Food is how we celebrate; food is how we commemorate.

Of course, there's nothing like a good food allergy or two to make us rethink all that. Whether your childhood memories centered on Christmas stockings bulging with candy and nuts or potato latkes and matzoh brie laden with rich eggs; a towering birthday cake or the giddy excess of a Halloween goody bag—it is likely that you may not be able to create the exact same experience for your child. It can feel a little sad, but it's not a total loss. Rethinking isn't the same as doing without. And let's face it: it's not as if some holiday traditions couldn't stand a little tinkering and rethinking in the first place. Use your child's food allergies as the opportunity to keep what you like most, and discard the rest.

HALLOWEEN

For food-allergic children, Halloween is the holiday that can seem the hardest to manage—all those gooey treats and bags of candy flying thick and fast from all directions—so it seems the logical place to begin.

Luckily, for the three-and-under set, Halloween is fairly confined. If your child attends preschool or day care, there will likely be a party and perhaps an activity or two to deal with. You'll probably want to bake some safe cupcakes or a special batch of cookies for your child to bring in and share with the class. Little ones are delighted by the way things *look* almost more than the way they *taste*, so your standard recipe topped with orange icing (just add a little food coloring to the plain icing recipe) and with a few pieces of allowed candy should work just fine if you're pressed for time. (See chapter 16, "Recipes," for a few quick and easy cake and cookie ideas.) If you're feeling particularly adventurous, bake a sheet cake, spread with "black" frosting, and decorate with orange icing pumpkins or whatever scary scene your imagination conjures up.

Children with wheat or gluten sensitivity can have a special treat that you've baked, Jell-O Jigglers in Halloween shapes (use cookie cutters or buy the Halloween mold from Jell-O), or Chocolate Dixies (see the recipe in chapter 16) filled with orange pudding, allowed candy, or orange sherbet. Halloween plates and napkins also add a special touch.

Never underestimate the power of stickers and other small gifts for this age group. A Halloween goody bag consisting of some orange and green Play Doh (for making pumpkins, witches, and ghouls, of course), some Halloween stickers, an allowed bit of candy, and a little toy will thrill most two- and three-year-olds. Be sure to confide to your child that the treats the other kids are eating will be gone in a matter of minutes, but that his or her special goody bag will last for *weeks*. (A note of deep sympathy in your voice for those poor children whose second-rate treats will soon be gone never hurts, either.)

Remember that even the best, most caring teachers may need some gracious reminding that your child cannot eat *anything* that you have not read the label for and approved. Even candy that would logically seem to be "safe" may indeed contain milk, egg, soy, peanut, nut, or wheat. Lately, I've been seeing a lot of candy corn and jelly beans that contain peanut oil or are marked "may contain peanut traces." Egg whites show up fairly often on these labels, too. Assume nothing. Read the labels. Know that the "fun" size of certain candies may include some ingredients that aren't in the regular size. And be sure to remind your child's teacher that even handling these foods for an art project, let's say, is not safe for your child.

We allow Lucas to trade in all the candy he receives at holiday parties for safe treats or trinkets—plus a little something extra as acknowledgment of the delayed gratification.

In general, Halloween is pretty easy to sidestep for the youngest kids. Give them a cute costume, a pumpkin, some easy craft projects, and some yummy orange-colored treats, and they feel the whole occasion has been a raving success.

For this tender age group, if you can avoid trick-or-treating, so much the better. In our experience, it tends to overwhelm even the boldest of them, and keeping track of all those potentially disastrous goodies can try your nerve as well. But if you have older children, or if you just can't resist showing the neighbors how adorable your little one looks in costume, you'll have to go to plan B, known in our house as the Halloween Bait-and-Switch.

I thought of a couple of different plans, actually, before deciding to go with this one. My first thought was to knock on my neighbors' doors a few days before Halloween, hand them a specially marked bag filled with candy I had preapproved for Lucas, and ask them to hand it to him when he came by with his dad and older brother.

This plan would have probably worked. It may even work for some of you. *But*—and there's always a but—I thought it left a bit too much up to chance. Would everyone have remembered Lucas's special bag? (Food allergies are hard to keep in mind for anyone who isn't dealing with them on a daily basis.) With all good intentions, would one or two people have put a little something extra in it that they felt sure was OK? And would Lucas, already no fool at the age of three years and nine months, have quickly decided that getting a special bag wasn't really so special? There were a few too many variables for me.

We decided to go with a slightly more daring plan, but one that has worked out just fine.

The real fun in going trick-or-treating, we decided, is not in eating all the goodies, although that is certainly a fine and grand thing. The *real* fun is in holding out your bag and collecting handfuls of wonderful junk like everyone else. So with my husband in tow, and a firm admonition (which we give to both of our boys) *not to eat any candy at all* until he gets home, Lucas rings doorbells and collects all manner of treats like all the other kids on the block. (Wrapped treats only, of course. I would not feel comfortable with him even touching treats that may contain peanuts.) When he comes home, he hands his candy over to me (which I either hide or dispose of), and I hand him an identical-looking bag stuffed to the brim with candy that he *can* eat. He gets the illicit thrill of collecting Snickers bars and Paydays, and I get the security of knowing that every bite that goes into his mouth has the Mommy Seal of Approval.

Frankly, I wish I could put this one over on my older son, as well.

If your food-allergic child is under the age of four, and you have older children, you'll have to be extra vigilant about what they bring into the house during Halloween. It can be all too easy for an allergen-containing candy bar to come home in a backpack and be discovered by a marauding toddler. Discuss the problem with your older children, and decide on some house rules. If you are not comfortable having any "unsafe" candy at all in the house, you might want to enact a bait-and-switch here, too. Stock up on some candy that's appealing and safe for everyone, and offer to trade with your older kids. Out go the chocolate-covered peanuts; in come the licorice sticks.

Or, if you do allow allergenic treats, make a plan for keeping them contained. Our older son knows to hand over all treats as soon as he gets home; then we put them in a marked, sealed container high in the pantry. When he wants some of his special treats, he eats them at a separate table from Lucas, wipes down the table after eating, and immediately washes his hands. He's willing to do it because he knows that otherwise he couldn't have the treats at all. It's not a perfect situation, but so far, it's the best compromise we've been able to reach.

GET READY FOR THE WINTER HOLIDAY SEASON

The good news is that holiday meals, for the most part, are extremely forgiving. Even if your child has many food allergies—to milk, eggs, peanuts, and nuts, for example—you'll be able to get around most of them with just a tweak here and there. But before we get into that, let's make sure you're fully prepared for the next few months.

Over the holidays it's a given that you'll be busy, and that your regular schedule will be disrupted. You'll probably be spending more time than usual out and about, visiting with friends, or going to restaurants. That famous Boy Scout motto "Be prepared" has seldom held more meaning than at this time of year. Prepare a few weeks before your schedule starts heating up by:

- Cooking and freezing individual portions of meals your child enjoys. Bring a portion with you when your family is invited for dinner at someone else's home, and make life easier for everyone.
- Checking your medicine cabinet to make sure you have a good, fresh supply of any and all medication your child takes regularly. Be sure you have at least two good EpiPens if your child needs to have one available, and enough liquid antihistamine. The same goes for all allergy and asthma medicines if needed. Because this is the beginning of the cold and flu season (and the start of nasty weather for a good many of us), I always try to have good stores of children's pain reliever, an oral rehydration solution like Pedialyte, and the kind of cough syrup my doctor recommends.
- Drawing up your plan of attack. What's most important for you

to accomplish over the holidays? Is it baking cookies and treats for family and friends or cooking some festive meals? Is it family togetherness time? Doing some holiday crafts? Make a special date with your kids to do *your* favorite thing and mark it on your calendar.

Now you're ready!

HOLIDAY HELPS AND SUBSTITUTIONS

Holiday food is based on meat and fowl, root vegetables, wheat products, and sugar, making it pretty easy to get around the peanut, tree nut, milk, egg, and soy question. Of course, if pecan pie is what makes Thanksgiving dinner worth eating for you, and your child is allergic to nuts, there's no real way around it. Have your pie at a restaurant and be done with it. But for the most part, you can substitute ingredients without anyone being the wiser. Here are a few hints to get around the major obstacles.

- Have you always bought one of those turkeys with butter solution under the skin or basted your holiday bird in butter? A simple and delicious alternative is to brush the turkey with allowed vegetable oil, season to taste, and pour three cups of allowed chicken stock into the bottom of the pan before cooking. Baste the bird periodically with the stock as it roasts, covering the breast with aluminum foil if it gets too brown before the inside is fully cooked.
- Is eliminating eggs throwing a kink into your holiday baking? My mother-in-law shared the secrets of her oil-based pie crust with me three years ago, and I've never looked back. Not only is this recipe egg- and dairy-free; the dough is the easiest I have ever made, I get a tender crust every time, and it works for both sweet and savory dishes. See the recipe in chapter 16, where you'll also find recipes for wonderful cakes and cookies.
- Eliminating wheat and gluten from a Thanksgiving feast is easier than it seems. The two primary offenders—the stuffing and desserts—have delicious substitutes.

- Wild rice or brown rice makes a wonderful stuffing base. Make a pilaf with the rice, cubed carrots, mushrooms, onions, and peas. Bind with some sharp cheddar cheese, if permitted. Or forget the idea of stuffing altogether: just toss some cubed potatoes, parsnips, carrots, and onions in olive oil and bake at 400° in a roasting pan for at least an hour for a rich, earthy dish that's welcome at any cold-weather meal.

- Instead of confining your thinking to cakes and pies for dessert, consider warm fruit crumbles, puddings and custards, ice cream or fruit sorbet delights, homemade fudge, caramel popcorn balls, and oatmeal squares. Make a fun candy turkey with permitted candy corn and marshmallows held together with toothpicks.

CHRISTMAS AND HANUKKAH

If you've ever found yourself starting to panic the moment Thanksgiving weekend is over, you don't need me to tell you about holiday burnout. It's a curious affliction: we so dearly want to make the season special for our families that we run ourselves ragged until a most *un*-holiday-like spirit prevails. As one who has dipped her toe into the waters of holiday madness more than once, I can testify that it's not a pretty thing. Here's the good news: unless you are the kind of person who is truly gifted in the domestic arts *and* who takes a bone-deep pleasure in their practice (be honest here), you might find that the so-called limitations imposed by allergy-free cooking and baking are actually rather freeing.

For example: Some years ago, after trying with extremely limited success to bake sheets of milk-free, egg-free gingerbread for a gingerbread house, I decided to take the path of least resistance and use milk-free, egg-free graham crackers instead. I have never looked back. For the past three years, the holiday season in our house has been ushered in with the purchase of three large boxes of graham crackers, as many bags of colorful, safe candies as we can find, and a fresh box of food coloring. I whip up a big batch of frosting, mix in food coloring, and turn on our corniest Christmas CDs while my two boys happily construct A-frame Christmas villages using the frosting as mortar and the candies as decorations. You can make or build whatever you like: Christmas trees, menorahs, stick-figure people, vehicles, or just tasty treats. Relax and be creative.

If your child can't have wheat, use allowed candy and thick frosting as bricks-and-mortar to build whatever structures or designs you like. Peppermint sticks can serve as logs; round candies can be wheels. Make a sled on candy cane runners. Build a snowman out of marshmallows and toothpicks. Make homemade fudge.

If your child can have ice cream, you can make an ice cream man. Simply place a gingerbread man cookie mold onto a plate, fill with softened ice cream, decorate however you choose, and return to the freezer. After at least an hour, remove the ice cream man from the freezer, run a knife around the edges of the mold, and lift as carefully as you can.

If your family celebrates Hanukkah and your child can't have eggs, you can grate a little cheese into the potato latkes to help them hold together. If milk is out of the question, too, try some bread crumbs and oil. If push comes to shove, you *can* just drop little well-rounded mounds of egg-free latkes into the hot oil. They won't hold together as well, but they will be delicious just the same.

BIRTHDAYS

Of all the special occasions in a child's year, his or her birthday is number one. It's number one for us parents, too, of course—I can't possibly be the only mother who blinks back tears as her child blows out the candles.

Although I've done my share of birthday parties at children's museums, play spaces, petting zoos, and the like, there's nothing like a birthday party at home to keep everyone relaxed. (OK, ten or more children under the age of five running wild through your house is not exactly relaxing, but it's still pretty darn good allergy control.) If your child can have wheat, you can bake a safe cake. If your child has to avoid wheat and gluten, you can serve make-your-own ice cream sundaes. If milk, eggs, *and* wheat are a problem, you can serve Chocolate Dixies (see the recipe in chapter 16) with your choice of filling. You can certainly bring any of these special foods to party places as well. They're just not as controlled a situation.

If you've read other sections of this book already, you'll know that it's my position—a conservative one, but not without warrant—to strictly avoid bakery products if your child is seriously allergic to peanuts, nuts, milk, or eggs. The reason for this is that bakeries run all their cakes, cookies, and pie fillings through the same equipment and frequently use the same bowls to mix batters without cleaning them out first. One can assume that cross-contamination is not just a possibility but a probability. The only way to be safe is to bake your own. Which is a natural segue into our next topic:

Other Children's Birthdays

Birthday parties come a close second behind eating in restaurants as food allergy stressors. You've got lots of kids, someone else's house, and all sorts of unidentified food objects floating around. Frequently adding to the stress is the attitude of the mother in charge, who may be either overly solicitous to the point of embarrassment or so casual about your child's food allergies that you feel you have no choice but to watch your child like a hawk throughout the proceeding.

With food allergies, as with football, the best defense is a good offense.

Even if you already know and have a friendly relationship with the mother issuing the invitation, it wouldn't hurt to sweetly remind her of your child's food allergies when you call to RSVP. After all, she doesn't live with them day in and day out the way you do. Even the most well-meaning moms may think nothing of serving peanut butter, for example, to everyone else and making a special sandwich for your child. What they don't realize is that just having all that peanut butter around is more risk than most moms of peanut-allergic children feel comfortable with. (And, as my friend Stacy found out the hard way, the birthday mom may use the same knife to cut your child's sandwich as she did to cut the peanut butter sandwiches. One

EpiPen injection and E.R. visit later, Stacy swore to always bring her son's food with him to parties.)

It's always important to find out what food will be served at the party, so that you can bring the closest approximation for your child. And of course, always bring your child his or her own portion of cake. Just bake a sheet cake or cupcakes every few months, spread on frosting, and freeze. You'll have cake at hand at a moment's notice.

Party bags, like Halloween goody bags, are another bone of contention. If at all possible, ask the party mom to leave the candy out of your child's bag, and bring some of your own allowed candy to put in it. If you feel too awkward asking, or if your child manages to nab another child's bag by mistake, be firm about not allowing any candy that does not have an ingredients label—but by all means offer an allowed replacement.

One of the issues that eventually arises is whether to stay at the party or just drop off your child and leave. Most young children *want* you to stay with them in unfamiliar surroundings, and you are probably more comfortable staying as well. As they mature, however, it can get more problematic.

If your child's allergies are severe enough to require epinephrine, you really should not leave him or her at a party without giving the party mom your emergency bag of epinephrine and antihistamine, plus instructions on when and how to use them. Assuming you've been careful and your child is careful, the need probably won't arise. However, it's the nature of accidents that no one expects them to happen. Needless to say, this is a big responsibility for another mom to undertake, even with the understanding that the odds of her actually having to give your child an injection are slim to none. (On top of the responsibility she's already assuming by having so many children at her house.) She would certainly not be outside the bounds of decency to refuse. In fact, it's better for her to honestly refuse the responsibility than to accept it lightly.

I've always found this situation—the handing off of my child to someone who is well meaning but has no long-term investment in him—to be the trickiest of all. It's not that I lack faith in the person, but that I lack faith in the variables. As anyone who's been dealing with a food-allergic child for a certain amount of time knows, keeping that child safe requires a lot more than just thinking ahead in a straight line. You have to think sideways, upside down, and at right angles, too. It takes effort, it takes experience, and it takes practice.

So far, I have always stayed at Lucas's parties because he is still young enough to want me to, and because there are always three or four other mothers staying as well. In the future, however, I will probably treat parties like swimming lessons: I'll drop him off and bring a good book to read in the car while I wait.

If you can spare the time to do it, you may find it useful to keep a holiday journal of solutions you've come up with and ideas that didn't quite work out, so that you don't have to reinvent the wheel every year. At the time, it always seems that we'll remember our successes, but a year is a long time. You may forget where you found a certain recipe or even what you served that got such rave reviews. You can jot down ideas as they come to you and clip interesting recipes from newspapers or magazines. Make it your own family's sourcebook. You can use a looseleaf binder, a folder, a spiral notebook, or even a recipe card box—whatever works for you. If you can get yourself into the habit of squirreling away a good idea here and a new recipe there, you'll soon find yourself with a treasure trove of resources.

21

TRAVELING WITH FOOD ALLERGIES

Whether your planned trip is short or long, traveling with food allergies requires pretty much the same degree of preparation. It has occurred to me on more than one occasion, as I ruefully surveyed the contents of my car trunk, that with all the gear I'm lugging I could just as easily be going to Paris as making a three-hour trip on the highway. But away from home is away from home: your pantry and medicine cabinet are just as inaccessible whether you're eating at a roadside McDonald's or a marvelous little boîte on the Left Bank.

As with all matters related to living with food allergy, careful planning and building a cooperative network are the keys to a successful travel experience wherever your travels lead. So the moral of this section is: load up your trunk and unload a little stress.

DAY TRIPS BY CAR

Truth be told, even before we knew about Lucas's food allergies I was never one of those cheerful, sporty moms who could fill up the car with kids, large dogs, and sporting equipment and take off on a two-hour trip with nary a juice box in sight. Nonetheless, I did cherish a fantasy of someday being that way. It was one of the many child-rearing fantasies I've bid adieu to over the past few years. (Remember the one about never blowing your stack with your kids? Good-bye!)

The fact is, traveling successfully with a food-allergic child requires planning. And we're not just talking about some well-chosen snack foods tucked into the trunk, with high hopes of an amenable restaurant beckoning a few miles up the highway. You need plan A, plan B, and (if your child has ever experienced an anaphylactic reaction) an emergency plan.

Like any new approach, the first few times are work. Give yourself enough uninterrupted time to do things properly. I've always found that the best time to plan out an upcoming trip (and by trip, I mean any time we're at least an hour away from home for the better part of the day) is right after the kids' bedtimes, when I've still got enough efficient-mother impetus going to resist the lure of the channel changer. I grab a yellow lined pad, sit at my kitchen counter, and work out what meals and snacks I need to cover, what medications I may need, and what I need to pack. Putting it all down on paper helps me calm the chatter in my head, and keeps me on track the next day when the whirlwind of activity, otherwise known as daily life with my two sons, threatens to blow me off course.

By now you know that my mind-set is always "*plan* for emergencies instead of *worrying* about emergencies." If I feel that I've covered just about anything that can go wrong—uncooperative restaurants or a server who just doesn't seem to be on the ball (this happens all too often, I'm afraid), poor menu choices, an asthma episode that arrives out of the blue, or even a serious allergic reaction—I don't have to think about it anymore. Living with the daily stress of constant vigilance takes its toll on all of us. Whatever we *can* do to reduce that stress, we *should* do.

So accept the fact that you'll be packing a cooler. It's your insurance. It's a lot easier to pack a cooler with acceptable foods than it is to wrangle with restaurant staff or have your child settle for a seriously subpar meal. (We have visited restaurants across the country where the only two things Lucas could safely eat were a hot dog—no bun—and ketchup. It happens.)

If your child has asthma or has had an allergic reaction requiring medication, accept the fact that you'll be packing medications. It's a lot easier to pack a meds bag than it is to start looking for an emergency room. And you should always have emergency meds with you in any case, even if you're just going to the grocery store.

But let's start with the cooler.

If your goal is to have your child eat restaurant food, make that your Plan A, but understand that you may be thrown a curve ball. Once Lucas grew out of his allergies to dairy and tomato (but not egg or peanut), we thought we'd always have pizza or spaghetti with tomato sauce to fall back on when we were eating out. Not so. On one vacation in Florida, over half of the restaurants informed us that egg was, indeed, an ingredient in their pizza crust, and most featured egg in their pasta as well. (A popular pizza restaurant at home in Connecticut uses peanut oil in its *sauce*.) French fries frequently contain wheat, egg, or nut ingredients. Hamburgers or hot dogs may contain just about anything. What's more, cross-contamination of foods is virtually unavoidable in many restaurant situations.

That being said, understand that the meal you pack in your cooler—the meal that in your mind is just for emergencies—may easily wind up being the meal your child eats.

Plan your cooler with that thought in mind. Eating out of the cooler may be plan B, but it doesn't have to taste that way. You're not limited to sandwiches. Even the least-responsive restaurants will nuke something for you if you explain your situation. So haul out that Tupperware and fill it up. I've packed cooked hamburgers on an acceptable bun, acceptable chicken nuggets, chicken drumsticks, thermoses filled with soup, lasagna, even one of Lucas's favorite casseroles. If your child loves hot dogs but can only eat certain brands, microwave the hot dogs in a dish filled with water, and pour the hot dogs plus the hot water into a thermos. They will stay hot and delicious for hours. Pack a bun and you're done.

My peak moment in packing-for-travel came when we took Lucas to his grandfather's retirement luncheon at a chic Italian restaurant.

At the time, Lucas was allergic to just about everything, but I managed to produce a reasonable facsimile of Osso Bucco (no butter, no tomato, no wine), which we called Luk-o Bucco, for my husband's birthday the week before. Our waiter whisked my Tupperware into the kitchen and returned with a steaming, fragrant plate. Lucas looked around, saw everyone else eating a meal that looked just like his on a plate just like his, and polished the whole thing off with a smile.

Grapes and raisins always travel well. If your child enjoys raw vegetables, pack an assortment in a water-filled container to keep them fresh and tasty. Don't skimp on the extras if that's what your child likes; pickles and chips are a big asset to any meal in our house.

Give some real thought to dessert. It is, after all, your child's favorite part of the meal, unless you've managed to achieve some level of parenting the rest of us have not. And desserts in particular are tricky in restaurants. If your child has wheat, egg, soy, milk, peanut, or tree nut allergies, you should avoid baked goods altogether. Even frozen desserts, unless well labeled, are suspect. Eggs are a common ingredient in premium ice creams and sherbets, and many carry a cross-contamination warning. ("May contain nut traces," for example.) Of course, many restaurant desserts come with no labeling information at all. On more than a few occasions we have sent a well-meaning waiter into the kitchen to read an ice cream label, only to be told that the container simply said "vanilla." In those cases, a restaurant dessert is simply out of the question.

It's always a nice thing for your child to have some special foods for special occasions. I keep individual portions of Wacky Cake (the recipe is in chapter 16) in the freezer and break them out only for birthday parties and restaurant outings. Individual bags of acceptable snacks—ingredient-approved pretzels, popcorn, crackers, or chips—feel more glamorous to my kids than a plastic bag of stuff. All that excess packaging isn't good for the physical environment, but it sure helps our emotional environment. I try to save candy for special outings and parties too. At the end of a meal, a lollipop and a bag of gummy creatures lasts a nice long time and really feels like a treat.

If your child has a favorite drink, by all means pack that as well. The only time we allow Lucas to have soda is in a restaurant, so he inevitably starts talking about his Sprite in the car on the way there. If you have a younger child, or if you just have higher nutritional standards than I do, pack the preferred juice. Restaurants don't always have apple juice available, and the orange juice is likely to have pulp in it. (Not popular at our house.)

In brief, plan the contents of your cooler as if that's the only food your child can eat for the duration of the trip. It may very well be.

When it comes to packing meds, particularly if your child has environmental allergies and/or asthma and you're traveling an hour or more away from home, I vote for packing everything. It's not as if you'll have to be carrying it, after all, and you can have the security of never being caught short. Think of your car as "home base."

Many parents, myself included, have found that it's actually easier to keep a packed bag of all your child's medications all the time, and to take the meds from the bag as you need them rather from an already-crowded medicine cabinet.

This works on a number of levels. For one thing, you don't run as great a risk of picking up the wrong medicine by mistake—selecting the amber bottle of your husband's prescription-strength cough medicine, say, instead of the same-color bottle of your child's Prelone for a severe asthma episode. All of the meds in your child's bag are for that child alone, and they're all in one place. Just pick it up and go.

You also get a better sense of what is getting used up, and what expiration dates are coming up, when you have all the meds in front of you every day.

When Lucas was still using a nebulizer to treat his asthma (for those lucky asthma-free families out there, a nebulizer is a fairly large, noisy, compressed-air machine that turns liquid medicine into a mist for inhaling), I packed it in a rectangular, nylon bag that had a few roomy zippered compartments. Some medicines—the albuterol solution and ampules of Intal—rode in the nebulizer, right in the same compartment with the machine's hose. Other medicines (bronchosaline solution, allergy medications, children's Tylenol, and PediaPred, an oral steroid) I zipped into a storage-size baggie and rested on top of the machine. I put an index card stating what the medicines were, the correct dosage, and when and how often to take each in the baggie with them. EpiPen and Benadryl went into a zippered compartment. (I always carry those two in my purse as well.) Forewarned is forearmed, and we were armed to the teeth. But I never worry when I travel (at least no more than usual), and you don't have to, either.

LONGER TRIPS WITHIN THE UNITED STATES

When it comes to taking a special trip, most children will be more interested in the amusements, hotel pool, or people they're spending time with than in what they'll be eating. Traveling, for young children at least, is not the gourmet experience we grown-ups may eagerly anticipate. Most children are happy with the simple food they enjoy at home, and can understand the fun part of the trip will be the experience, not the ice cream. But as parents, we want them to enjoy it all, and that often means actively seeking out the places where our children can enjoy a normal meal.

For our family, if that means returning to the same restaurant every day for lunch, as we did two summers in a row at Walt Disney World, so be it. By the end of our stay, we'd made friends with all the waitresses and eaten more hamburgers, french fries, milk shakes, and parfaits than we'd eaten in the entire previous year, but we were relaxed and happy with every bite. I think it's important for young children that their parents make managing food issues look simple, not unlike trapeze artists. As a spectator, you can't help sometimes thinking, "Gee, I could probably do that." But as a rational adult, you know that countless hours of training went into giving that impression.

Whenever you're traveling outside your region, the following pointers can make life easier and safer.

- Brands that you rely on at home may have a different formulation in another part of the country. Although you should *always* get R.E.A.L and Read Every and All Labels, please pay special attention when you're away from home.

• If you're staying in a hotel, whenever possible choose accommodations that have a kitchenette or at least a mini-refrigerator. If this isn't possible, consider bringing along a large ice chest. Our routine, which has saved everyone a good deal of worry and frustration, is to do some light grocery shopping as soon as we've arrived at our destination and unpacked our bags. Most places you'll travel to will have at least a convenience store or corner deli nearby. Being able to count on our supply of fresh fruit, cereal, bread, sandwich meat and cheese, and assorted snack foods and special goodies makes everyone feel more in control at mealtimes and gives us a pleasant degree of flexibility.

• Bring along your child's school lunch box, complete with cold pack and thermos. Pack it full of safe foods your child enjoys and zip it into a backpack with a few extra treats each day. Although it happens rarely, we have encountered restaurants where there was virtually nothing on the menu that was both safe and appealing for our food-allergic little one. One restaurant chain, which seemed like a sure thing at first glance, turned out to use both peanut oil and egg in the pizza, eggs in the hamburger and hot dog rolls, and peanut oil in its french fries and potato chips. I will never forget the sight of Lucas being served one plain hot dog on a big white plate, which is why I have never been caught unprepared again.

• Avoid situations where guests serve themselves from a buffet. Even if a few dishes are safe for your child to eat, serving spoons from other foods will no doubt come into contact with them, raising the issue of cross-contamination. If your child is only allergic to peanuts and tree nuts, buffet-style breakfasts may be safe, provided you have checked out the ingredients of all the food on offer with the chef. In general, the more gourmet the restaurant fancies itself to be, the greater the risk that you'll encounter a hidden allergen. ("A little hazelnut butter on your french toast, Madame?")

• To be filed under the category of "any port in a storm": some of the fast-food franchises that have become a fixture on every highway now offer printed sheets listing the ingredients in all of their offerings. If you don't see them at your favorite establishment, just ask.

You may well find that your child can safely eat a number of the menu items. What's more, as of this book's writing, the Burger King Web site allows you to read the ingredients of every Burger King item from your home computer before you even set out on your journey. We can only hope that other restaurants will follow suit! While I'm hardly advocating a steady diet of fast food, it's an unavoidable truth that most children love it. (And I must confess to some previously undetected warm and fuzzy feelings toward establishments that let my child feel like all the other kids in the junk-food department.)

• If you are traveling to visit friends or family, consider shipping some favorite foods to their house before you arrive. While most food allergies can be easily accommodated across the country, special needs such as bread for a wheat-allergic child or soy milk for a dairy-allergic child may be problematic, particularly in more remote areas. Sending a "care package" in advance not only assures you of having exactly what your child likes and needs, it saves you the hassle of extra luggage.

FLYING WITH FOOD ALLERGIES

The farther away from home you travel, the greater chance there is that you'll choose to fly. But it's the rare parent of *any* child who can board an airplane without at least some anxiety; keeping most children happy, comfortable, and occupied during a flight of any length over an hour is a challenge that cannot be understated. And as always, when you throw food allergies into the mix, everything becomes a bit more complicated.

If your child is allergic to peanuts, traveling by air can feel a bit like being held prisoner in a hostile nation. For generations, we Americans have been conditioned to associate flying with cute little pouches of salted peanuts. Like Pavlov's dogs, when we see the drinks cart come rolling down the aisle, our mouths start watering for those crunchy, tasty treats. Never mind that while we're on the ground peanuts are available to us at any hour of the day, any day of the week; when we're on the plane, we don't merely want them—we feel it's our right to have them.

Needless to say, if you are the parent of a peanut-allergic child, you want to limit your child's exposure to peanuts as much possible. This is simply common sense: when hundreds of bags of peanuts are all opened at the same time, there is a certain amount of peanut protein released into the air. Some peanut-allergic children will have no problem with this whatsoever, provided they don't eat or even mouth any peanuts themselves. Some will experience allergy symptoms such as a runny nose, redness of the skin, or coughing. Extremely hypersensitive children—about 1 percent of children who are peanut-allergic—may wheeze or show other signs of distress. Fortunately, there are no reported instances of a child dying on a plane who did not actually eat some quantity of peanut, no matter how minute.

As recently as four years ago, flying with a peanut-allergic child could all too often degenerate into a highly unsettling situation. We had several flights back then, and I thought I was prepared. From my Food Allergy Network (FAN) newsletters I had learned that it was possible to alert airlines ahead of time that a peanut-allergic child would be on a certain flight, and request that an alternate snack such as pretzels be served. Many families reported great success with this method.

Not us.

Although we always called ahead a few days before the scheduled flight and again on the actual day of the flight—both times receiving reassurances that no peanuts would be served—no one apparently ever thought to inform the crew. And thereupon followed a string of experiences that were almost Kafka-esque in their bizarreness. Most notable was the flight attendant who, upon being oh-so-gently asked if she could possibly substitute another snack for peanuts on her flight, looked me dead in the eye, told me she had never in her fifteen years of flying heard of anyone being allergic to peanuts, and loudly suggested that I needed some serious psychiatric help. I suggested to her that the pilot might not be too pleased about being asked to make an emergency landing, and would she please consult with him on that. (I didn't necessarily think that this would be the case, but what really burned me up was that during our entire interaction I was looking over her shoulder at a big basket of pretzels.) And yes, they did serve the pretzels instead of peanuts, but I could not wait to get off that plane.

Happily, in the past year some airlines have gone peanut-free, and many others have become more sensitive to the needs of their peanut-allergic passengers. Flight attendants have become noticeably more understanding, although they may only hand out pretzels in the five aisles ahead of and five aisles behind you.

Unfortunately, one or two airline holdouts will adamantly refuse to accommodate you, and go so far as to forswear any responsibility if you fly with them. I have heard of several occasions where the airline has actually refused to let peanut-allergic children fly on its planes unless their parents signed documents absolving the airline of all responsibility in the event of an accident and agreed to pay the costs incurred in an emergency landing. (In all cases the parents signed the forms, figuring they'd fight it out later if they had to. And in all cases the child was just fine, although the trip cannot have been pleasant.) This is clearly an extreme reaction, and one would hope that the probability of encountering a similar one will be slim-to-none.

But airline policies change all the time. Your best bet is to call the airline of your choice as far ahead as you can and determine where it stands. If you don't feel comfortable, choose another airline if possible. And of course, even if the airline graciously complies with your request, it cannot control the food that other passengers bring on board. If your child is hypersensitive to peanuts, understand that other parents may have packed peanut butter sandwiches for their children to eat on board, which is their right. If those kids are seated near you, it's obviously a less-than-ideal situation, but it's not a genuinely life-threatening one, either. Besides, there's really no way around it.

If your child is one of those rare people who experiences distress from merely smelling peanuts, consult with your doctor before boarding a plane.

One word about airline meals: don't. The margin for error is simply too great, and no one should have to undertake treating a reaction at 35,000 feet. It takes just a few minutes to pack fresh fruit, allowed snacks, and either a hot meal in a thermos or sandwiches. Pack twice as much as you think you'll need to cover any delays you may experience. Then relax. A side benefit to packing your own provisions is that your child can eat when he or she gets hungry. No waiting for meals, no fussing about food that may be less than satisfactory. (Although most young children, to their elders' dismay, adore airplane food.) A steady stream of allowed goodies makes the time go by faster, too.

Although you certainly don't have to do this, I always try to pack a meal for myself too, so Lucas doesn't feel that he's the only one who has to have a special meal. Yogurt, bagels, fruit, cheese, and cookies are easy to pack and preferable (to me at least) to whatever the airline chooses to bestow upon us.

Many parents have expressed concern about placing their child in an environment where so many peanut fragments have been living for so long. They've got a point there; we've all been on planes where the housekeeping standards have been less than stellar. Even the cleanest planes have years' worth of microscopic peanut crumbs mashed into their carpeting, upholstery, and ventilation systems. Luckily, a lot of peanut-allergic children only experience nuisance reactions at most—runny noses and itching or reddened skin—to the aircraft environment. Many allergists recommend giving a peanut-allergic child a dose of the preferred antihistamine one half hour before boarding, which seems to do the trick. Ask yours what tack you should take.

As you've gathered by now, I'm a firm believer in the portable medicine cabinet. The list that follows encompasses what you should have on hand if you are packing for a child with food allergies and asthma (the most meds-heavy situation). If your child does not have asthma, the list still stands but for the asthma medications.

- Two EpiPens and a full bottle of liquid antihistamine, with measuring cap
- A rescue inhaler (for asthma)

- A bottle of liquid steroid (for asthma emergencies)
- A wide variety of nonperishable snacks, all of which your child has eaten before. (To be on the super-safe side, because there is a remote possibility that any given brand of packaged food may be mislabeled or contain undeclared ingredients by mistake, you might want to make sure that your child has had some crackers from the cracker box, some cookies from the cookie box, etc., a few days before you leave, while you're still on terra firma.)
- Water, juice, and a few lollipops, to make take-off and landing easier on the ears
- Lots of favored reading material and activities, to keep your child from getting bored and to provide a distraction if you need to treat asthma or another reaction
- A beloved doll or stuffed animal from home, for the same reasons
- A copy of your emergency action plan, with doctors' phone numbers

If your child relies on a nebulizer to treat moderate-to-severe asthma, you should know that there is no place on board a plane to plug one in. If the asthma can flare up without warning and he or she is too young to use a portable inhaler, Dr. Alejandra Gurtman, medical director of the Travel Health Program at Mount Sinai Hospital in New York, suggests that you may want to consider investing in a battery-operated nebulizer. They're quite expensive, running over $400, but if you fly fairly often or are planning an overseas flight the expense may be worth it. If you know of another family who could use it, perhaps you could go in on the purchase together. Personally, I would consider it money well spent to be able to quickly and effectively treat just one asthma episode that might have otherwise turned into a problem. The peace-of-mind factor is priceless. On a long trip, your asthmatic child will also probably be more comfortable if you pack his or her own pillow and a light blanket for the plane, reducing the dust mite exposure as much as possible.

Dr. Gurtman also recommends bringing along a peak-flow meter for lung capacity. A peak-flow meter lets you measure how well your child is breathing long before nasty symptoms like coughing and wheezing begin. Most asthmatic children will show a decline in lung capacity for at least a day or two before an actual asthma episode begins, which allows you to begin treatment before symptoms progress to the point of distress. Most children over the age of four can learn to use one.

The last but perhaps most important item to keep in mind when you're planning a trip is simply this: take a good, hard look at how healthy (or not) your child has been over the past month. If several allergic reactions, asthma episodes, or other health problems have occurred, you may want to give your plans some careful thought. Do you feel prepared to handle, on your own, any similar problems that may come up far from home? Do you want to?

I'm certainly not suggesting that a long-anticipated trip to Walt Disney World should be iced because of a few wheezing episodes. But if your child has really been struggling recently, his or her health won't suddenly improve the minute the Magic Kingdom is in sight. And not only will an under-the-weather child miss out on a lot of the fun, there will be a real drain on your energy, too. On the other hand, Orlando has excellent health facilities should you need them, and you won't find more pleasant, helpful people than the Walt Disney World "cast." You may decide to take your trip as scheduled but cut back on some of the activity. If you can tell your child is tiring out by 11:30 A.M., you can always go back to your hotel for lunch, a leisurely dip in the pool, and perhaps a nap before setting out again.

Similarly, if the trip is a long-anticipated family reunion, just try to put as many safeguards into place as possible before you go: ask your relatives to help you find a good local allergist who can be called upon if necessary; make sure you know the route to the local emergency room; and try to tailor the schedule to your child's comfort level.

If, for whatever reason, you find that you really must put your travel plans on hold, it's best to be tactful with your child. Stress that the trip isn't canceled, just postponed (if that is indeed the case). I wouldn't even be above fabricating a different reason for the postponement, such as really bad weather in the area or the hotel having to close temporarily for renovations. The point is to not put undue emphasis on the child's health. I don't think any of us want our children growing up to think that the world revolves around their health issues (although it can certainly sometimes seem as if our parental world does). We also don't want to unduly alarm them, as in "if we're canceling our trip, I must be really sick." A cheerful, matter-of-fact approach is best. There will be disappointment, of course, but your optimistic frame of mind and reassurance that the trip will indeed come to pass can go a long way.

TRAVELING ABROAD

Once you venture outside the United States, the rules change quite a bit. Foods are not labeled the same way, legal requirements regarding labeling are different, and the language barrier can seem formidable. But as always, the Food Allergy Network, working in cooperation with the Information Centre for Food Hypersensitivity (LIVO), has done the advance work for you. Contact FAN at (800) 929-4040 for the most up-to-date information on labeling rules (which change fairly frequently), how to reach emergency medical services, in-country organizations devoted to food allergies, plus translations for more than twenty commonly used allergy terms in these countries:

Belgium
Canada
Denmark
France
Germany
Hungary
Iceland
Luxembourg
Netherlands
Poland
Spain
Sweden
United Kingdom (England, Wales, Scotland, and Northern Ireland)

. . .

If you are planning a family trip abroad, FAN also has an excellent pamphlet, titled *Travel Guide: Tips for Traveling with Food Allergy*, that belongs in every parent's carry-on bag. The information it contains is vital. For instance, did you know that vegetable oils are manufactured differently abroad and may contain allergenic protein? While a soy-allergic child may safely consume soybean oil in the United States, outside the country soybean oil may very well cause a reaction. If at all possible, order the brochure a good six weeks in advance of your trip. That way, you can organize the information you need and make whatever calls you need to make without feeling that you're cutting corners due to time pressure.

And remember that wherever you travel, the same rules apply regarding avoiding possible cross-contamination and hidden allergens. Vacation time is not the time to let down your guard. But once you have the facts and draw up an eating plan, your family's trip to a foreign country can be every bit as safe, inspiring, and memorable as any other family's. Enjoy it!

22

OFF TO SCHOOL

THE PRESCHOOL YEARS

There are generally two ways parents learn of a child's food allergy: before preschool, and at preschool. (You'd be surprised to learn just how many little ones have their first reaction in a classroom.) If you fall into the former category, you've no doubt chosen or will choose your child's preschool or day care center with safety in mind. If your child had his or her first reaction at school, you've got to play a little catch-up. Either way, the general guidelines for keeping your child safe and happy are the same.

You should know that children with life-threatening food allergies are protected by federal laws prohibiting discrimination on the basis of disability. Unfortunately, this does not mean that you'll find an informed awareness of food allergies and willingness to comply with safety issues at every preschool or day care center. Just a few short years ago when I was beginning to look at preschools for Lucas, I was treated to reactions from school directors that ran the gamut from positive, calm, and completely in control to near-hysteria at the thought of having responsibility for a peanut-allergic child.

Today, I think it would be rare to find a well-established preschool or day care facility that does not have at least *some* experience in taking care of a child with food allergies. However, its attitude will be a factor in your decision. If you are getting resistance from the preschool or day care center of your choice, or if you're just picking up signals that make you uneasy, you will have to ask yourself some questions. How important is it to you for your child to attend this particular program? If the program is your first choice because of the fine music or art activities it offers, but you have other choices you feel good about, you might consider going with another program and enrolling your child in separate art or music classes. If it is extremely important for your child to attend a particular program because it's the only one that offers the hours you need or some other concrete factor, are you willing to put some real time and effort into working with the staff to maximize your child's safety—and their goodwill toward your family? I truly believe that you can turn just about anyone around—and in the long run, you'll all be glad you did—but it would be unfair to underestimate the work involved.

Resistance is an interesting beast. It can seem slight but be maddeningly strong. Or it can seem overpowering but collapse with a few friendly, intelligent words. If you've decided to deal with it, your best first step is to try to figure out where it's coming from.

You know this, but I'll tell you again anyway: most resistance comes from fear. Happily, that fear isn't generally of litigation, although the directors of some schools will say it is. They may say that the only way your child can attend their program is if you sign a liability waiver, which is just plain foolish. For one thing, if they have agreed to take care of your child, that's what they must do. Certainly, they'd be held liable if a child with no food allergies quietly slipped out of the classroom, crossed the street, and got hit by a car. That's a crime of inattention. If a jar of peanut butter is left open in the middle of the table and your peanut-allergic child decides to try some, that's a crime of inattention too. The second thing about liability waivers is that they've been thrown out of court when they are used to deny a person his or her rights under the law. And your food-allergic child has a right under the law to be kept safe from allergens.

Your bottom line on liability waivers should be "don't insult my intelligence." I will trust you to put that in as tactful yet clear a way as you can. Understand, however, that accidents can occur at even the most vigilant nursery schools and day care centers, the same as they can at a restaurant, at a relative's house, or at home. Just as a child's chin can hit a perfectly safe chair in just the right way to require stitches (as happened to us twice with our older son, both times the day before class pictures were taken), schools cannot control every molecule of a child's environment. Like you and I, they can only do the best they can.

Most genuine resistance comes from fear of the unknown. People who have never had to learn the symptoms of an allergic reaction or have never used an EpiPen may have "awfulized" these situations in their heads. And let's face it, we parents are not entirely innocent in this regard. When your child has a scary reaction, it can be tempting to overdramatize it in the telling. We may do it without even realizing it. Everyone at some point has heard about a child "blowing up like a balloon" or a similar happenstance, when in fact many of those reactions were not nearly as horrific as the description would suggest. (Some, of course, *were* truly awful.) If we want people to react calmly and matter-of-factly when we tell them about our child's food allergies, we need to act that way, too. Some people may resist taking responsibility for a child with food allergies because the picture in their heads is so horrendous. The only way to find out if that's the issue is to ask.

Here's where it gets sticky, of course. If you gently ask, "What do you think will happen if my daughter eats _____?" and the school director says, "Well, I'm afraid she will stop breathing and die," the school director may have a point if your daughter has life-threatening allergies. The same, however, could be said of any child who begins to choke on food or a small object. And the school director may not know how relatively simple it is to keep your daughter safe or how straightforward it is to treat a reaction that is just beginning.

Again, the best defense is a good offense. If you have all your ducks in a row before you even begin to contact schools—action plans, meds, list of safeguards—*you* will feel calmer and more confident, which will translate to the school director. An optimistic, can-do attitude is the best armor you can wear if you suspect a small battle may be in the offing. How much nicer to be prepared with firm resolve and a smile in your voice—"I know that people may feel a little nervous with Marie at the beginning, but that won't last long. I have everything you need to make things run smoothly and easily, and I'll always be available when you need me"—than to feel defeated and depressed if you receive a less-than-warm welcome.

Family Day Care

Family day care (where your child is taken care of in another person's home) is another matter entirely. Some family day care providers will feel that they can't take on the responsibility, and that's that. Others will have experience with food allergies and feel confident that they can keep your child safe, or will be happy to go through the training required. There are many family day care providers who take a great deal of professional pride in their skills and are eager to add to them.

With family day care, there are both pluses and minuses. On the positive side, you have a commitment from the person directly in charge of your child, as opposed to an amenable school director but a nervous teacher. A family day care provider can set any standards she wants. (If she says no tree nuts come into her home, no one can argue about that.) There are also fewer children involved, so there's less food coming and going. On the negative side, you are asking her to police her own home. If her children eat and enjoy foods that your child is allergic to, how will she arrange her own kitchen to keep your child safe? You are also dealing with someone who essentially has no backup. How will she take care of the other children if your child has an allergic crisis? (And how will she take care of yours in the same situation?)

Family day care can be an ideal situation for a food-allergic child. It can also be less than ideal. Ask plenty of questions, listen to your intuition, and make your decision.

Safety First

Whether your child is already enrolled in a preschool or day care center, or you're just beginning to look at options, make sure you've answered all the following questions.

1. Is there an up-to-date action plan, with fresh medication, easily accessible? Does everyone know where it is and how to use it?

2. Does everyone who will be taking care of your child know what the symptoms of an allergic reaction are, and know that any physical symptoms your child reports after eating need to be taken seriously?

3. Is your child's food allergy posted where everyone entering the classroom can plainly see it? A brightly colored sign outside the door that reads "No nuts, please! We are a nut-free classroom!" is a useful warning for all visitors. Inside the classroom, there will need to be a sign posted saying which child has the allergies, and where the child's action plan and meds are located, in the event of an emergency.

4. Is there a plan in place for informing *substitute* teachers of your child's food allergy, and what to do in an emergency?

5. Do you have good communication with the teachers regarding snacks and birthday treats? Has someone been assigned to read all ingredients labels, or have you worked out a system where you supply your child's snack? Does the teacher give you a day's warning before an in-class birthday party, so you can pack your child a safe treat? You might decide to always pack your child's own treat and leave one less detail up to chance.

6. If your child is severely allergic to peanuts, have you worked out a peanut-free zone in the classroom and made sure that children who eat peanut butter have their hands thoroughly washed with soap and water after eating? Are tables wiped down, too?

7. Is there a number at which you or a trusted caregiver can be reached *at all times*? Many parents of food-allergic children carry beepers for this purpose. I carry a cell phone that's always on during school hours and recharge it at night.

8. Do the parents of the other children in your child's class know about your child's food allergy? Some people prefer to let the school inform other parents about their child's food allergy; others prefer to send a personal letter themselves. Either way, you and the school will have to put your heads together about the letter's content. Some pre-school classrooms ban peanut butter altogether when one child has an allergy, while others make arrangements to keep the allergic child safe. It would be hard to ban milk or products containing eggs. If you are writing your own letter, show it to the school director and your child's teachers before sending it out.

9. Have you made provisions for field trips? Your child's medication and action plan must always be brought along, whether the trip is a walk to the neighborhood post office or a long bus ride to the zoo.

Because preschoolers are such hands-on learners, it wouldn't hurt to also have a discussion with your child's teacher about the materials she plans to use in class. Counting pumpkin seeds, M&M's, or sunflower seeds may be a good way to teach number concepts, but to a peanut- or seed-allergic child, even handling these foods may be dangerous. (My friend Stacy found out that her son was anaphylactic to peanuts when he was making a bird feeder—a pinecone rolled in peanut butter and then in sunflower seeds—in his nursery school. Just the peanut butter on his hands was enough to trigger a major reaction.) Peanut shells are also frequently used in art projects but should not be touched by peanut-allergic children. Plastic yogurt containers make great paint jars, but they must be completely and thoroughly washed out to protect milk-allergic children, as do milk cartons, pudding cups, and any other dairy containers.

A Day Care Center Director's Perspective

Heather Klein is executive director of the Wilton Children's Center, a day care facility that is licensed by the State of Connecticut Board of Health and fully accredited by the National Association for the Education of Young Children (NAEYC), which sets federal guidelines for high-quality child care. Recently she shared some thoughts with me on how she and her staff have successfully managed food allergies and sensitivities among their young charges over the years. Parental attitude is key, Ms. Klein noted. Her suggestions to parents are to:

• Approach the school in a spirit of cooperation. Although most day care centers and nursery schools will make a strong effort to keep *every* food-allergic child safe, there's no denying that staff will go the extra mile for a family that presents concerns in a reasonable manner and expresses their appreciation clearly and often. Avoid being pushy.

• Provide as much information as possible about trigger foods, symptoms that may indicate an allergic reaction in progress, and a step-by-step accounting of what to do in an emergency. A clear, detailed action plan is a must.

• Acknowledge that while the school can and should control what food is available in the classrooms, the school cannot control all of what comes in via children's coat pockets, with visitors, or with siblings. It's simply impossible to police everyone at all times. One always hopes that families will make a conscious effort to keep another child safe, but there probably will be at least one slip-up over the course of a school year: the toddler brother with a leftover bit of peanut butter toast clenched in his fist, or the baby-sitter who absent-mindedly puts her Snickers bar down on a table to help a child put on a coat. The child care center needs to make every possible effort to keep the allergic child safe, but there are an astonishing number of variables. The parents must realize that guaranteeing an absolutely, 100 percent allergen-free environment at every moment is simply not possible.

• Understand how much work goes on behind the scenes to keep a food-allergic child safe and the wheels of progress greased. Ms. Klein recalls having to deal with families who very much resented being asked not to send peanut butter sandwiches into school because of a highly peanut-allergic child in the class. One mother in particular expressed her displeasure loudly and often, and it became a regular feature of Ms. Klein's week to deal with this woman's complaints.

At one point she even volunteered to take one family, who insisted that their child would not touch any food other than peanut butter, to the local Stop & Shop to point out all the other delicious options available. (A desperation measure that she was not taken up on.) She also had to deal with teachers who resented and were frightened by the added responsibility of caring for a food-allergic child. Neither instance is at all unusual. Although, appropriately, she shared none of this with the food-allergic children's families, the astute ones suspected how much effort she was putting forth and thanked her often. It made a difference.

Heather Klein's recommendations for directors of preschools and day care centers who may be dealing with a food-allergic child for the first time are to:

• Communicate thoroughly and often with the staff of the *whole school* about the child's food allergies, not just the teachers of the class involved. It's important for *all* staff members to be alert to the signs and symptoms that may indicate a child is having an allergic reaction, for a variety of reasons: The regular classroom teacher may be having an off day or an exceptionally busy day and may not notice symptoms right away herself; the reaction may occur when the regular teacher is on break or is out sick; the regular teacher, although trained to handle an allergic emergency, may panic in a crisis and need backup help. In the best of all possible worlds, the staff should be able to act as one to protect the food-allergic child.

• Following the same logic, mandate EpiPen training for *all* staff members. Licensed facilities should already have a connection with their local health department, which should be able to either provide in-service training or steer your school to the proper provider. If, for whatever reason, that is not possible, local doctors or nurses can provide the same service. Training generally does not take more than one hour, and virtually all staff members find it much easier than they expected.

• Communicate thoroughly and often with any other groups who may use the preschool facility, to ensure that they don't bring in unsafe foods. Stress how vitally important this is, and also ask that they wipe down all tables with soap and water at the end of each session. In my own personal experience, the same YMCA classroom that Lucas enjoyed a few hours in each week as a two-year-old was also used as an after-school place for older children. One morning I brought Lucas into the classroom to find unshelled peanuts lying on the rug. Barely breathing, I picked them up, then made an inch-by-inch inspection of the rest of the room. Needless to say, thorough inspection of the premises became a regular feature of my visits to that center, and with no offers of cooperation forthcoming, we looked elsewhere for a preschool program.

• Make sure all parents of children enrolled in the allergic child's class understand that food allergies need to be taken seriously. Be prepared with suggestions for lunch and snack options that other children have enjoyed.

• Thoroughly review the foods that may be offered to children during the course of the school day. Most preschools feature morning snacks, and day care centers feature snacks twice a day. Make sure that more than one staff member knows how to read a label for food allergy, and ask for the parents' input whenever necessary.

• Put a system in place for storing epinephrine, and make sure that everyone understands the limitations intrinsic in its storage (for example, it cannot be refrigerated and cannot sit out in the hot sun). Teach staff members how to check if epinephrine is still fresh, and make sure it is checked regularly. Many schools use a portable locked box to store the epinephrine, but be sure that the location of the key is known to all! The locked box must also accompany the child on all field trips.

On the plus side, having a classmate with food allergies offers a living lesson in compassion and caring to all the other children in a class. Even children as young as three seem to understand how serious an issue a food allergy is. We've had many, many moms call and tell us how pleased they were that their child adamantly refused to bring certain favorite foods to school because it wouldn't be safe for Lucas. And when Lucas outgrew his allergies to milk and eggs, every child in the class celebrated. A short video available from the Food Allergy Network, *Alexander, the Elephant Who Couldn't Eat Peanuts*, is a charming and informative way to teach little ones about food allergy. It can be ordered directly from FAN. (See the section on ordering materials from FAN that appears later in this chapter.)

There's no doubt that food allergies add an extra layer of concern when it comes to away-from-home situations for our little ones. But try to keep them just that: a *layer*. While your child's safety has to come first, making new friends, having fun, and feeling successful in a group situation are vitally important, too. I knew I was going overboard on the allergy thing when Lucas's playground "pick-up" line became "Can you eat peanuts?" Try to avoid talking about the food allergy in front of your child as much as possible. While the topic certainly shouldn't seem off-limits, it shouldn't be the defining characteristic of your child, either. I know how hard this can be; I've been pigeonholed as "the allergy mom" for many years now, and although I do enjoy sharing information with other parents, it can get a bit old. I don't think I've yet achieved the perfect balance—having other parents aware enough of Lucas's allergy to keep him safe, but not so aware that his allergy isn't the first thing they think of when they think of him. I'm working on it.

ELEMENTARY SCHOOL

Compared with the relative safety of preschool, parents find they have less control over their child's elementary school environment. Classes are generally much larger, but only one teacher is in charge. And while most preschools are small, privately run enterprises that can change their policies to suit the children enrolled at the time, public elementary schools are less flexible. In elementary school there are more variables all around: more kids, more staff, more activities, more opportunities for play dates with classmates you may not know as well. Your child is truly beginning life in the great big world.

It's a marvelous journey. And if you let them, your greatest friends and allies on that journey will be the school staff: your child's teachers, principals, and school nurses.

The best way to get off on a good foot is by planning ahead. If you know what elementary school your child will be attending in September, don't wait until the first day of school to distribute action plans and meds. You can start laying the groundwork as early as April or May.

Classroom Teachers

If your child's teacher has not had a food-allergic child in her class before, she may feel apprehensive at first. Even if she *has* dealt with food allergies, she may feel a bit stressed out. That's OK—being responsible for a food-allergic child *is* a bigger responsibility than most teachers bargain for, especially when the allergy is life threatening. And frankly, I'd rather my child have a slightly nervous (and therefore, more cautious) teacher than one who is a little too carefree. The most important point to keep in mind is that you are on the same team. Give the teacher your full support. Let her know how much you appreciate her efforts on your child's behalf, and encourage her to communicate all of her feelings—positive *and* negative—with you. That's the only way you'll learn what works and what doesn't. The goal here is to work out the best, most efficient ways of keeping your child happy, learning, and safe.

You can make the teacher's job much easier (and provide your child with a safer environment) by following these guidelines:

If at all possible, arrange a time before the school year begins to sit down and have a brief face-to-face meeting. Use this time to explain your child's allergy, how it was handled in preschool, and what you will do to make sure everything runs as smoothly as possible in the classroom—helping out at class parties or contributing baked goods, for instance; or coming in to the class to speak about food allergy. Emphasize to the teacher that you are available to her at all times should she have any questions, and you are open to her input in terms of what will work and what won't. This is a nice opportunity to lay the foundation for what should be a friendly, mutually respectful, and honest relationship.

Before the first day of school, provide the teacher with:

1. A complete description of your child's allergy, including symptoms and a list of foods and ingredients to avoid

2. An action plan and medication, also to be given to the school nurse

3. A sizable quantity and good selection of safe snacks—acceptable candy, salty snacks, packaged cookies, and the like—to be given to your child when his or her classmates are enjoying a similar treat

4. A letter that can be sent home to the parents of your child's classmates, explaining your child's allergy and asking for their cooperation

5. A list of practical safety guidelines that should include ways to avoid cross-contamination, the necessity of avoiding food-trading at lunch and snack time, a "code word" your child can use if he or she thinks a reaction is starting, and the need for careful supervision at parties and other food-related occasions

Not until my older son came home from kindergarten with chocolate on his face every day for a week did I realize that a lot of extracurricular eating goes on at school these days. Many teachers are accustomed to rewarding students with a food treat: a pizza party if the class reads 100 books in a month, let's say; or ice cream cone gift certificates as holiday gifts for all. Some teachers may even have traditions they've established: they may bake special Valentine's Day cookies for their class every year, or bring in a cake for an end-of-year celebration. Food may be a part of learning: teachers may show the class how to churn milk into butter as part of a social studies lesson, or bring in ethnic foods to highlight the study of a particular country. Parents from different cultures may bring in special foods to teach the class how their family celebrates the holidays. To the oh-so-slightly paranoid parents of a food-allergic child, it can seem like a regular food fest every week of the year.

Happily, this veritable tidal wave of food is not as uncontrollable as it may appear. It just requires a little rethinking. Food is certainly an easy and fun way to celebrate, but there are lots of other options for every holiday. Parties that feature a craft activity plus goody bags filled with inexpensive treats, such as stickers, special pencils, and tiny toys, are lots of fun, too.

Most teachers are quite open to the idea of food-free parties—after all, they're the ones who have to maintain some semblance of peace and order in the classroom after their students have had their fill of cake, cookies, and candy. Parents might offer a bit more resistance. As with everything else, the chemistry of that particular group and your child's particular allergy will lead the way to a solution all of you can live with. Some groups of parents just seem to bend over backward to be helpful, while others have their backs up the minute they hear a food-allergic child is in their child's class. Most fall somewhere in between, with some exceptionally helpful and compassionate parents, many caring and concerned parents, and a few parents who plainly resent any outside control over what their child brings into the classroom. It's all a matter of give-and-take, with just one nonnegotiable: your child must be as safe during a party as during the regular school day. That means that everyone coming into your child's classroom, especially during a party, must know about your child's food allergy and understand what is involved in terms of safety issues.

The School Nurse

If you are as lucky as we are, your child's school nurse is part angel, part health care professional, with a sprinkling of earth mother thrown in for good measure. It's the nature of the job. If you are cheerfully willing and able to handle everything from bruises, wet pants, and "the throw-ups" to asthma, migraines, spiking fevers, and medical emergencies all in the course of a day's work, you are a very special person indeed.

School nurses are an invaluable resource to all of us with food-allergic children, but we must be wary of laying too big a burden at their feet. Yes, they are usually the most qualified people on staff to handle a medical crisis, but they are not, and should not, be the only ones capable of acting on your child's behalf should the need arise. (And unfortunately, at some rural locations and even some private schools a school nurse must divide her time between two or more buildings.) It goes without saying that the school nurse must have your child's action plan, meds, and any special instructions including your emergency phone number. But if your child has an allergic reaction in a classroom far from her office or on the playground, a teacher or playground attendant may be the one handling at least the first stage of your child's treatment. It's important for *everyone* who will be in contact with your child—not just the nurse—to know what to do in an emergency.

With the school nurse's help and cooperation, some schools stage mock "fire drills" in which they pretend that a food-allergic child is having a reaction in the classroom or on the playground. This kind of exercise can be helpful in more than a few ways: learning how long it really does take for the teacher to unlock the lockbox and administer the child's medication; how long it truly takes to get to the nurse's office (or how long it takes the nurse to get to the child) when an emergency situation is under way; even finding out what may have slipped through the cracks in terms of preparedness.

Because communication is the key to keeping your child safe in school, keeping a running dialogue going with your child's school nurse—at least one phone call or note per term—can certainly make everyone feel safer and more comfortable. Ask her if she has any suggestions and be sure to regularly express your appreciation for her attention and concern.

HELPFUL PROGRAMS AND MATERIALS

Materials from FAN to Help Ease the Transition

Help is at hand! Here is a partial list of materials that can be ordered from the Food Allergy Network (FAN) to ease the transition from home to preschool or elementary school. Booklets are generally priced from $5 to $8, videos from $15 to $20. School programs are priced at approximately $75. Call FAN at (800) 929-4040 to order or for more information.

- *Commonly Asked Questions about Food Allergies* (booklet)
- *Just One Little Bite Can Hurt! Important Facts about Anaphylaxis* (booklet and video)
- *Understanding Food Labels* (booklet)
- *Off to School with Food Allergies, Parent/Teacher Set* (two-booklet set plus teacher's guide)
- *Students with Food Allergies: What Do the Laws Say?* (booklet)
- *The School Food Allergy Program* (video, 100-page binder, poster, and EpiPen trainer)
- *The Childcare and Preschool Guide to Managing Food Allergies* (two videos, binder, EpiPen trainer, "How to Read a Label" cards, and poster)
- *Food Allergy Awareness* (poster)
- *Be a Pal* (poster)
- *Alexander, the Elephant Who Couldn't Eat Peanuts* (video)
- *Alexander, the Elephant Who Couldn't Eat Peanuts* (coloring book)
- *Let's Party: Themes, Tips, and Recipes* (book)

Introducing PAL: Protect a Life from Food Allergies

The Food Allergy Network (FAN) has developed a new program called PAL, aimed at all school-age children. PAL is free of cost to all schools who want to participate. The purpose of PAL is to get peers involved in keeping food-allergic children safe. And when a child involved in PAL helps out in a noteworthy way—intercepts an allergen-containing goody, let's say, or recognizes that a friend is having a reaction and goes to get help—that child receives a PAL Hero Award. The premises of PAL are simple enough for even elementary school students to understand, yet are vitally important for everyone to know:

- Never take food allergies lightly.
- Don't share your food with food-allergic friends.

- Wash hands after eating.
- Ask what your friends are allergic to and help them avoid it.
- If an allergic schoolmate becomes ill, get help immediately!

For more information on PAL and other programs, contact the Food Allergy Network at (800) 929-4040.

TO BAN OR NOT TO BAN?

In response to parental pressure and concerns about their own liability, some preschools, private schools, and public schools have instituted a "peanut ban." In effect, they are attempting to create a peanut-free zone within the school. No peanuts, peanut butter, or any other food products containing peanuts are technically allowed within the walls of the school, on the school buses, or on the playground.

Other schools, particularly at the preschool level, have instituted partial bans. Peanut products are banned within the peanut-allergic child's classroom, but children in other classrooms are free to eat them. This is generally done in recognition of the fact that little people who eat peanut butter have a tendency to leave tiny dabs of the stuff on tables, blocks, and toys, setting up a dangerous situation for the allergic child.

Needless to say, banning is a loaded topic. Parents who are in favor of banning peanuts can cite numerous instances in which their child was exposed or was almost exposed to enough peanut in the environment to cause a serious reaction. Parents who oppose banning can cite the rights of the other children, as well as a host of complications that banning may create.

The Food Allergy Network (FAN) does not support a schoolwide peanut ban for a variety of reasons. Chief among them is that a peanut ban creates a false sense of security. In reality, enforcing a ban like this is virtually impossible. Peanuts and peanut protein are in so many different foods that each parent in the school system would have to be both highly educated in food allergy and completely motivated to be compliant with the ban for it to succeed. And what about the children who are highly allergic to other foods? A drop of spilled milk can spell as much danger to a highly milk-allergic child as a dab of peanut butter does to a peanut-allergic child.

Although often undertaken in good faith, a ban can make peanut-allergic children feel even more different than they may have felt already, which breeds an unhealthy self-consciousness.

What's more, a ban is bound to engender resentment among parents. Human nature being what it is, a few parents will embrace a ban as a lesson in compassion, many will feel irritated but comply in good faith, and an inevitable handful will be outraged enough to openly express their sense of injustice and try to subvert the ban however they can. Instead of neutral bystanders, they have become the enemy, creating a more dangerous situation for the allergic child than may have previously existed.

As parents of food-allergic children, we are all too aware that the moment our children leave our homes we are to a certain extent dependent on "the kindness of strangers": the cafeteria aid who tactfully sees to it that our daughter is seated in a "buffer zone" with friends who aren't eating peanut butter; the school bus driver who decides to hand out stickers instead of candy for holiday treats; the recess monitor who sees a few hives on our son's face and gently pulls him aside to further assess the situation. Goodwill, cooperation, and education are the keys to keeping food-allergic children safe, but none can flourish in an atmosphere tinged with rancor.

Complete and accurate ingredients listings, and education on avoiding allergic reactions, recognizing a reaction in progress, and treating it the proper way are the best safeguards for school-age children.

23

YOUR SCHOOL-AGE CHILD'S
EMOTIONAL WELL-BEING

When your food-allergic child leaves the gentle preschool world behind, everyone's lives change. While that first transition from toddler to preschooler was certainly a milestone, the transition from preschooler to kindergartener or elementary school student is much more dramatic. Suddenly you don't know about every part of your child's day (which was usually helpfully supplied by the teacher if your child was not so forthcoming) or every child in the class. Part of that is simple logistics: your child's class size may be considerably larger now, and if your child rides the school bus, you don't have the daily rhythm of drop-offs and pick-ups that once helped you develop relationships with your child's classmates and their parents or caregivers. You're simply not as connected to the ebb and flow of your child's day as you may have been.

To an extent, that's how it should be. It's what independence is about after all, and as good parents we know that's something to be encouraged. But when your child has health concerns that require steady attention and care, it's harder than usual to find the balance between freedom and control that gives your child enough space to grow in, and lets you feel confident about food-safety issues at the same time. What's more, once your child is in elementary school and beyond, common childhood issues such as feeling different, being teased or even bullied, and feeling anxious, depressed, or ashamed take on a whole new resonance when a chronic condition such as food allergy is attached.

Being at best a seat-of-the-pants home psychologist with my own boys, I enlisted the aid of Claudia Manis, M.A., a gifted and perceptive school psychologist at Hurlbutt Elementary School in Weston, Connecticut. In the twelve years that Claudia has been helping children with difficulties in their school or home lives, she has observed a great degree of similarity in the issues faced by children with any ongoing health concern, from diabetes to asthma to seizure disorders to food allergy. The everyday challenges of childhood—feeling different, being teased, feeling left out—aren't any different for children with health concerns than those without, but they can be magnified.

Just as adults often ask "why me?" when something bad happens, children can feel that having a food allergy is an unfair burden. That's certainly understandable (and as parents, we can't help agreeing in our hearts that it *is* unfair for our child to have to deal with this), but it isn't an attitude that bears encouraging. Dwelling on life's injustices isn't just unproductive; it's a skewed view of reality. If "fair" means having everything just the way we want it all of the time, life isn't fair for anyone, really: there's the neighborhood child who has to wear thick glasses or is unusually short; the classmates who must struggle to keep up in school; the children who long to be athletes but are always picked last for teams; the kids who can't seem to make friends or have to move a lot and start at a new school almost every year. Yes, there are those few children who seem to sail through life with nary a worry or problem, but they are the exceptions. In dozens of large and small ways every day, life "isn't fair" for all of us.

Up to a point, it's helpful to acknowledge your child's feelings of anger and frustration. Everyone feels the need to be truly heard, and none more so than children, who are frequently all too aware of their vulnerability and powerlessness. We all should encourage our children to speak freely and from the heart. But it's important to let our children know that while they have our love and understanding—and of course we wish that they did not have to deal with a food allergy—*we do not feel sorry for them*. Their food allergy is just a part of life that can be more or less easily worked around. A matter-of-fact attitude is the best possible defense against a child becoming overly fearful or even manipulative, using the food allergy (or asthma) as the trump card.

A few children can develop a sense of importance and specialness relating to their allergy that is just as daunting and damaging as those who feel sorry for themselves all the time. Usually, these are the children who have been fussed over, worried over, sheltered, and coddled way beyond what's necessary to keep them healthy and safe. Needless to say, as these children grow up, they will have trouble making friends and developing a sense of true self-esteem. What's more, an attitude like this can even be dangerous to a child's health. While most school-age children feel a natural compassion and sense of protectiveness toward the food-allergic child in their midst, a child who acts spoiled or insists upon special treatment all the time will very soon wear out that compassion and alienate the very people who matter most when it comes to having a happy school experience.

It's important to know that many young children, and even those as old as six or seven, may feel that they've done something bad to cause their food allergy. In a young child's magical inner world, just thinking something may cause it to happen (hence the fear and guilt many children feel when something bad happens to someone they're angry with). By the same token, if something is wrong with them, it stands to reason that it's because of something they thought or did. It's logical thinking in its own way: "I'm only punished when I'm bad; food allergy is a punishment, so I must have done something bad." The cues may be hard to pick up, but some children who are dealing with these feelings may act out or even become self-destructive. As parents, we need to do what we can to make clear to our children that their bodies—and many other peoples' bodies—are just this way. They did nothing to cause their food allergy, just as a boy who wears glasses did nothing to harm his vision, and a girl who has a big nose did nothing to make her face look that way.

The fact that the child did nothing to cause the food allergy, and can't do anything to make it go away, makes teasing a particularly tender topic. To be teased about the shirt you're wearing or the back-pack you're carrying is one thing, but to be teased about a condition that you not only have no control over but dislike as well can be very hard. Of course, children are teased all the time about their flaming red hair, their multitude of freckles, their small stature, or wide girth, but few parental alarm bells ring. We feel sympathetic, and we offer our child support, but we don't usually feel that our child is in real danger unless the teaser is a physically aggressive bully. What can set us on edge if our child is teased about a food allergy is the remote but nonetheless real possibility that the teaser may take things too far and expose our child to a truly life-threatening situation.

Happily, with young children and even those in the lower elementary school grades, being teased about a food allergy is generally not an issue, and only a handful of cases have been reported in which a food-allergic child was taunted to the point of danger, usually in the middle school years. And in terms of safety, there are usually plenty of adults around watching children fairly carefully at this age. But because young children usually don't have the forethought to avoid situations that may include teasing, and can't even really tell when teasing is about to turn ugly, they are usually shocked and dismayed when it happens at all.

It would be wonderful if we could all teach our children certain strategies to "immunize" them against being teased or feeling bad when they are. But just as teasing affects each child differently, there are no hard-and-fast rules to apply if and when your child is the chosen target.

The bottom line is that being teased means realizing that not everybody is nice. All of our children, food-allergic or not, need to understand that people who are dedicated teasers are people who are not happy with themselves, so they take those feelings out on others. But teasing hurts nonetheless, and the calm, sympathetic, and matter-of-fact reaction of adults is crucial to helping children regain their equilibrium. While we must certainly let children know that teasing is unacceptable, it never helps to blow teasing out of all proportion.

If a teacher or parent overreacts to standard-issue playground teasing, children are left to infer that teasing isn't just unpleasant—it's downright dangerous.

Because most young children are unprepared to deal with any amount of serious teasing on their own, they need to feel safe in telling adults about being teased without being branded a tattletale. But some children are too ashamed. Others are afraid of retaliation. Still others may feel that telling won't help, or worry that they won't be taken seriously. Whether or not children seek out an adult at school to confide in, they need to at least tell one of their parents if they're being teased. Psychologists agree that what's most important is not the level of teasing itself, but how children interpret the teasing and what they tell themselves about it. A child who can think "I hate it when Wendy says those things. She's just a meanie, and they're not at all true" is in a much better position than the one who thinks "She's right. I'm just a stupid kid who can't even eat a peanut butter sandwich, so of course people aren't going to want to play with me." The reality of life is we truly *can't* control what others feel and say. All we can do is control ourselves. And that is a teachable skill. Children really do believe what we tell them, so if the messages we are sending are positive and strong—"you showed such team spirit at your soccer game; you were such a good friend when you consoled Susan; you came up with such a creative solution when you figured out how to share the paints"—they will integrate those feelings into their own self-image. As parents, we can make all the difference in how our children interpret and respond to life's occasional unpleasantness.

When your child comes to you with distressing reports from the bus, lunchroom, or playground, the two of you can decide whether your child should confront the bully or just make peace with the situation. A direct approach is usually better, because most teasers and bullies, especially little ones, are all bluff. When they sit down together to discuss the problem, it's not unusual for the tables to be turned, with the bully turning into the child's protector. But if your child is extremely uncomfortable with confrontation, don't force it. An indirect approach can work, too. A teacher can confront the bully and explain that she's heard about the teasing. Sometimes it's possible for the children to be separated. Or you and your child may decide to do nothing at all, assuming the situation falls more under the category of annoying than misery inducing. So long as your child does not take the teasing personally and can maintain positive self-esteem throughout it all, there's no real harm done.

Occasionally, however, whether because of excessive teasing and feeling different, a bad reaction that was either very embarrassing or required a hospital stay, a good many more asthma episodes or eczema skin flares than usual, increased tension in the family, or a number of other reasons, even young children may become anxious or depressed. And what may be confusing to parents is that neither disorder always presents itself in a pattern that's immediately recognizable.

Most of us think of depressed children as sad children. We associate depression with listlessness, withdrawal, teariness, and a general blue lethargy that just doesn't go away. Certainly, children who act this way are sending a very clear signal that they are having an awfully rough time of things and may in fact be depressed. It's plain that these children need help. Not so obviously depressed are the children who suddenly become much more "hyper" and angry than usual. They may be having sleep issues, unexplainable bathroom accidents, or an unusual number of bad dreams. They may be acting far more aggressive than usual on the playground. They may have recently lost a number of friends due to their acting out. This kind of behavior is harder to read. It may be an exaggerated developmental hump or an indicator of some other problem. But it can be depression too. Anger and depression are closely linked.

Anxiety, on the other hand, can look like an attentional issue. The child simply can't concentrate and learn. But unlike ADD, anxiety is not a sensory processing problem. The anxious child is just too worried or nervous all the time to be able to attend. A child who is having a problem with anxiety (or depression for that matter) may not enjoy activities that were always a source of pleasure before. He or she may hold back from participating in group activities. A child who is feeling very anxious may develop phobias relating to food or eating, or related phobias such as a fear of going to school, riding the school bus, or being separated from the parent at any time. Anxious children may become compulsive and overcontrolling because they feel so out of control in their daily lives. They may become rigid about changes in their day, getting completely thrown off course if they can't have their favorite cereal for breakfast or wind up having a substitute teacher, because they feel so vulnerable. They can show an unusual amount of anger and react unpredictably to different situations.

If you are concerned that your child may be anxious or depressed, the defining question to ask yourself is: have I observed a marked negative change in my child's behavior that has lasted for over two or three weeks? If the answer is yes, it's time to get busy. Most young children have a hard time articulating why they are suddenly droopy and sullen when they were once cheerful and active. They'll say, "I don't want to play with my friends because I don't like them anymore," or "I don't want to go to school because it's boring." They can't say that the reason they don't want to play with their friends is that they don't feel like playing much at all these days, or that they don't want to go to school because just about everything but staying at a parent's side feels too unsafe and overwhelming right now.

Some children who are showing symptoms of anxiety or depression may just happen to be going through a particularly rough stage of life and will sort themselves out perfectly well with some extra patience, love, and understanding. But if you feel unusually concerned about your child, or your child's teacher or school guidance counselor expresses concern to you as well, your child may benefit from some professional help. Your pediatrician or school psychologist will be able to recommend qualified people who have experience in helping children through particularly trying times in their lives.

It would be wonderful if we all came into this world instinctively knowing how to best handle a crisis situation, or if we were routinely taught crisis management in grade school, but that's not our reality. A child who has a life-threatening food allergy (or any other serious health condition, for that matter) throws a family into crisis—sometimes for a few weeks, other times for years. There are steps we can put in place to manage the day-to-day details. But how we and our children react on a gut level to crisis is only partly within our control; some of us are hardwired to withstand great amounts of stress, whereas others can tolerate very little.

If your child is suffering from depression and anxiety, it is certainly worthwhile to make your lists and check them twice. Ask yourself honestly: Am I overanxious or sad myself? Am I overprotective or underprotective? Is there a high level of tension in the house? Are we all feeling a bit out of control? In a family, what affects one person affects us all. But understand that children may become anxious or depressed even in good family situations. We can safeguard them as best we can by setting a positive example, putting all systems in place to keep them safe, encouraging open communication, and offering plenty of love and support. In most cases, that's enough. The few children who are temperamentally prone to experiencing some emotional difficulties deserve and need our help, but they do not need our self-recrimination and self-blame.

Of course, the food-allergic child isn't the only one with an emotional burden to bear in a family. Siblings are deeply affected too. Whether they're aware of it or not, some siblings may feel guilty that their brother or sister has to observe rigid eating restrictions or else risk a serious reaction, while they can eat whatever they please. Others may feel resentful that the food-allergic child receives more attention and has special meals prepared for him or her. Some siblings may take on some of the parents' worry about the food-allergic child, whereas others will rebel and seem not to care at all. Often the feelings are all mixed up together.

"Why should I always have to worry about him? He never has to worry about me!" is a commonly heard sentiment from siblings of food-allergic children, and certainly an understandable one. It wouldn't be untoward for a parent to gently point out that everyone would do the same for him or her were the tables turned. Underneath the bluster, however, may be a brother or sister who is feeling truly oppressed by an atmosphere of tension. As parents, we must ask our children to observe precautions regarding food whenever they are home, but we can also ask them how we can make it easier for them. If there's something in particular that's really bothering them, we need to know. It's far easier and quicker in the long run to deal with the root cause of a negative feeling than continuously battle the difficult behavior the feeling engenders. What's more, there's almost always a way to work it out.

My older son, Dylan, missed going out to Chinese restaurants and eating certain kinds of candy the most. So now whenever I can, I take him out for lunch over the weekend. He picks the restaurant. We also try to arrange for him to spend time with his grandparents in the city, who are happy to take him restaurant hopping across Manhattan. The candy issue was even easier to resolve. When he brings home a party bag, we go through it and put all the "off-limits" candy on a high shelf. He may request this candy for dessert but must eat it in his room and wash his hands afterward. Play dates and overnights with friends, sleep-away camp, and school lunches all give him the opportunity to eat treats such as peanut butter, baked goods with nuts, and nut candies that we don't feel comfortable serving.

Removing the resentment and feeling of overresponsibility from siblings not only helps us have better relationships with all of our children, but also helps the siblings enjoy a better relationship with each other.

24

ANXIETY, ANGER, AND DEPRESSION

Over the past few years, I've received more than one phone message from a mom that goes something like this: "Hi, Marianne. You don't know me, but my name is Susan, and I was given your name by the school nurse. My son, Jack, is anaphylactic to peanuts, and let me tell you, the stress is absolutely *out of control* around here." I know that on a certain level most of the moms are exaggerating—their children are doing fine, all the right safeguards are in place, the home is being well run, and the mom has activities in her life that bring her pleasure. But on a deeper level, I know there's no exaggeration about it: the stress of caring for a child who can suffer life-threatening consequences from just the teeniest bit of the wrong food—and knowing it could happen at any time at all—can all too easily feel overwhelming. But what we call "stress" is more often than not a mixture of emotions. We say we feel anxious; we say we feel a little depressed; we may even say we feel angry. It's hard to tell where one feeling ends and another begins—or even what exactly it is we're really feeling.

Some parents, not worriers or brooders by nature, are able to incorporate this added pressure into their lives without everyone's anxiety levels rising accordingly. But for many of us—and I must count myself among them—it can indeed at times feel deeply uncomfortable to know that a precious child is vulnerable to great harm every time he or she eats.

If you are the kind of person, for example, who can brush off a series of small setbacks—your husband snapping at you for forgetting to run an errand, the blouse you had planned to wear coming back from the cleaners minus a button, and then your car not starting—with a shrug and a rueful sigh, then you probably won't be too easily unhinged by dealing with the day-to-day stresses of life with a food-allergic child. On the other hand, if you are the kind of person who can be easily thrown off stride by any small number of mishaps, life is probably going to be a bit harder for you because life is a bit harder on extra-sensitive people *all* the time. In other words, if your antennae are always up and vibrating a bit, they're just going to vibrate more when you introduce more stress.

It can be helpful for those of you who fall into this second category to understand that your uncomfortably intense reaction to your child's situation isn't some new and aberrant behavior that has sprung full-blown out of nowhere, but rather just a few ticks higher on the anxiety continuum you're living with already. The better you understand and accept how you react to stress, the easier you can be on yourself. This doesn't mean that you should just give in and let those highly anxious feelings flourish, but a pep talk to yourself—along the lines of "OK, Jennifer, you know that you tend to magnify things and worry about them, and that's just the way you are, but let's see if you can get a little perspective here"—might be in order.

What's more, put in its proper place and harnessed to some productive goals, stress needn't be all bad. For example:

There was a time, not so long ago, when I heard through the grapevine that some of the mothers of children in Lucas's class very much resented the fact that they were asked not to send peanut *treats*—such as peanut candies, peanut butter granola bars, peanut butter cookies—into the classroom. (Peanut butter sandwiches were gently discouraged but by no means forbidden, with the understanding that a peanut butter ban would pose a genuine hardship to those families whose kids wouldn't eat anything else.)

These moms were outraged that someone was "controlling" what they packed in their children's lunches. The fact that another child's life was at stake seemed to mean little or nothing to them.

My initial response was shock. How could women who had precious children of their own be so self-absorbed, so uncaring? Moments later, I got scared: what if these moms had so much of their identities invested in not being "controlled" that they would pack peanut butter sandwiches every single day for their kids? What if they would even try to sneak peanut butter products into the classroom out of sheer defiance?

Then I got angry.

Dr. Elinor Greenberg urges us to think of our emotions as a "tool kit" and to think of normal anger as one of our very best tools. The physical purpose of anger is to fill us with chemicals that allow us to be stronger, braver, and take action: the "fight" part of the famous "fight or flight" response. She likens it to a chemical "pill" that gives us more energy as it takes away our fear. And with that fearless energy, you can do things you may have thought unthinkable or, at the very least, deeply uncomfortable. All of a sudden, you can pleasantly yet firmly confront a fellow parent or a teacher over issues of safety; write a carefully worded letter of complaint to the chief executive of an airline or restaurant chain that was disrespectful of your child's special needs; what have you.

Conversely, if you're angry at yourself for a justified reason—perhaps you didn't speak up when your best friend prepared foods that were dangerous for your child while your family was at her house, or perhaps it was *you* who didn't read a label and your child suffered a reaction—you can use that energy to make the necessary changes. Change can be very hard. You *need* an extra hit of energy from somewhere. Good, focused, productive anger can be a good place to find it.

By the way, I used my anger at the "uncontrollable" moms to arrange for a chance to speak in front of all the parents at Back to School Night. In as gentle a way as possible, I told the story of Lucas's first peanut reaction—how red and swollen his skin was, how labored his breathing was, how we slipped and skidded over the icy streets on our way to the E.R., how I sang him nursery rhymes in the backseat fearing they might be the last sounds he would hear. I tried to make it personal and real to them. I wanted them to put *their* children in my story.

The meeting was a success. I didn't hear any more rumblings, at least from that particular group of moms, for the rest of the year. That doesn't mean there weren't any, of course. What I learned from that experience is that there are always going to be people who mistake your reasonable efforts to protect your child as efforts to control *them*, and who will react accordingly.

While anger is a tool of fearlessness and energy, anxiety is a tool of vigilance. It's a warning from our body that we have something to be afraid of, something to watch out for. Clearly, when you have a child with serious food allergies, a certain measure of anxiety serves a useful purpose. It warns us to carefully scrutinize ingredients labels, carry epinephrine and Benadryl wherever we go, draw up emergency action plans, and make ourselves well known to school nurses. Anxiety warns us to check, beware, take action. Anxiety insists that we remain alert, reminding us that not reading ingredients or not checking with the waitress "just this one time" may have devastating results.

Anxiety is a signal that you must attend to something in your environment. But for all too many of us, the signal still keeps coming through loud and clear long after we've restructured our pantries and our lives to fully accommodate our child's needs. If you ever find yourself in this position—or you find that you're pretty much *always* caught in an anxiety holding pattern—you need to do a rational check.

Ask yourself: Have I taken all the appropriate action that it's necessary for me to take? (This doesn't include what you wish *other* people would do, because to a great extent other people's actions are truly beyond our control.) Have I put in place as many mechanisms as I can to protect my child? Is there something in the back of my mind that I haven't done? Am I truly doing everything I can? If the answer to each question is an unequivocal yes, your anxiety has served its useful purpose. It's time to give yourself the permission to stop feeling anxious.

Easier said than done, you say? Don't I know it, especially because none of us could have claimed stress-free lives *before* we were dealing with food allergies. That one extra stressor can be all it takes to move us past the pleasantly heightened states of keyed-up and on-our-toes to stress overdrive. But I've found several useful strategies for keeping anxiety down to a faint hum. The first, and easiest, is to make one big master list of everything I'm doing to keep Lucas safe, from reading lists of ingredients at least twice, to staying in touch with the school nurse and keeping track of epinephrine expiration dates. When I see it on paper, I'm able to convince myself that I really do have all the bases covered. Another useful tool is the bimonthly newsletter published by the Food Allergy Network (FAN). Anne Munoz-Furlong, FAN's founder, packs every issue with practical information and tips on keeping kids safe. If she includes information I haven't considered before, I add it to my master list. If she talks about safeguards that have been second nature to me for years, I get to feel like Master of the Allergy Universe for a few deeply satisfying and all-too-brief minutes.

It's possible, however, that the reason you are still feeling anxious is because there are still some loose ends you haven't attended to. If you ask your rational mind why you are feeling so anxious, you might become aware of something you really should have done—talked to the school nurse's assistant, let's say, or put a plan in place

---

Things I Have to Do Today: Breathe In, Breathe Out

When we can control our breathing, we can also begin to control our anxiety. The reason is biological: when we are anxious, our heart rate speeds up. Taking long, slow breaths brings our heart rate down and makes us feel calmer almost immediately. When you are beginning to feel anxious, try breathing in slowly through your nose to a count of five and out through your mouth to a count of ten. Within four or five breaths you'll probably begin to feel your heart slowing down and will feel a bit calmer.

to notify any substitute teachers of your child's allergy. There may be some tasks that you find difficult or unpleasant, and therefore have been putting them off: ordering an EpiPen trainer from FAN and practicing with it, for instance, or sending out a letter to the parents of your child's preschool classmates, telling them how severe your child's allergy is and asking their cooperation in keeping your child safe. In this case, you're getting a lingering anxiety signal because it's not yet appropriate for the signal to turn off. Procrastination is anxiety's best friend.

If despite all your best efforts—food carefully scrutinized, medications packed, list of all the precautions you're taking checked and approved—you still find that you have an uncomfortably high level of anxiety about your child's food allergy, perhaps what you need to attend to is not in the outer environment but within yourself. Ask yourself: if a red button suddenly appeared in front of me that would magically shut off my anxiety, would I push it? Don't be surprised if your first response is *no*! Many people fear that if they give up their vigilance for even a moment, they will make a mistake that has awful consequences for their child. They feel a basic lack of trust in themselves and the world in general. After all, what kind of world is it where a child can die from one bite of birthday cake?

Another reason for persistent anxiety is as a cover-up for other emotions. What feelings have you been experiencing that are too uncomfortable to confront directly? Ask yourself: if I weren't feeling anxious right now, what would I be feeling? See what comes up.

Many people find that under their anxiety there's a lot of anger, both rational and irrational. And in the hallowed tradition of "you always hurt the one you love," some people deal with the anger they feel by focusing on their mate's imperfections. If you're a woman, you're more likely to call this deep anger anxiety and say you're anxious about your mate not doing the right thing.

In fact, it may turn out that you feel perfectly justifiable anger at your spouse for not helping out as much as he or she could, or for downplaying the seriousness of your child's health risks. You need to talk about it, either between yourselves or with a counselor, and work out a more equitable way of sharing the responsibility. Not only does your child's health depend upon it, the anxiety won't go away until you do, and your marriage will suffer.

Then again, your spouse may be doing everything he or she can, but you still feel overburdened and resentful. Again—talk about it in as friendly a way as possible, using "I" sentences: "I feel upset when you do this" instead of "You always do this!" Explain that you are aware that your anger is not wholly justified, but you don't want to keep feeling this way and you need your spouse's help. Perhaps your spouse is being wonderful with your child but has withdrawn some emotional support from you. You feel abandoned and alone. Perhaps you are not comfortable with the role you play in managing your child's allergy. (See chapter 26, "Emotional Leaders and Task Leaders.") Perhaps you somehow assumed that your spouse would play the leading role in a situation such as this, and even dividing the responsibility feels difficult for you. Clearly, the two of you will have to come to some arrangement, but you'll also have to make some inner adjustments.

You may feel anger at the child, beloved as he or she is, for making life so difficult at times. You may feel anger at parents or grandparents who have food allergies or other allergies themselves, for the genetic material they bequeathed you. You may feel anger at the parents of "normal" kids: why did they, instead of you, get an easy child? You may feel anger at God, anger at the makers of all allergen-containing products, anger at the world. At the core of this kind of anger is a feeling of helplessness. It's not often in our safe, comfortable, rational lives that we have to deal with the consequences of events that are truly out of our control.

In ancient times, people had an easy explanation: if something was wrong with you or your child, you must have done something to anger the gods. People accepted that the gods were easily angered, frequently for no discernable reason. And given that most of us have a little something we feel a bit guilty about, an explanation for the gods' wrath is never too far behind. Of course, if we can anger the gods, we can also propitiate them, which gives us back a certain measure of control.

Granted, there's a certain amount of irrational anger that's a natural consequence of being a modern American, with our great sense of national entitlement. Since all things are supposed to be possible in our country, almost all of us assume, misguided or not, that if we do the right thing our lives will go smoothly. So we study in school, get good jobs, work hard, make some sacrifices to reach our goals, marry a good spouse, the works. According to our internal logic, we've done our part, so success is guaranteed. Of course, underneath it all we know that life doesn't always work out the way we planned. But logic has nothing to do with anger. The fact remains that your dreams for your child and your family have been, if not completely destroyed, at least seriously damaged—and you're furious.

If you find this irrational sort of anger hiding beneath your anxiety, acknowledge it and try to get some help. Anger is a tough row to hoe, and you may not be able to handle it all by yourself. For some people, support groups are very valuable, especially when you're feeling a bit isolated because no one else you know is going through the same thing as you. Even your dearest friends will get bored with hearing the details of your child's reactions and restrictions, and may even get annoyed with you for "obsessing" or "overreacting." (Or worse, you may get the same reaction as I did from one beloved friend, who told me that when she's having a really bad day with her kids, she reminds herself that I have it harder every single day. Hmm. Thanks for sharing.) I guarantee that you'll have an eager audience in a food-allergy group—if only because they want *you* to listen with rapt attention when it's *their* turn to speak. The point is to get together with some people who make it safe for you to be yourself and air your feelings. Chances are, there will be at least one or two others in the group who are feeling or who have felt the exact same way. Somehow, hearing irrational statements out of someone else's mouth can help you let go of the same feelings. They sound ludicrous! Or, conversely, being shown great empathy for those feelings can help you heal.

If you've tried support groups and feel that you weren't sufficiently helped by them, a little therapy might be in order. By *therapy*, I don't mean the lengthy kind of complete personality restructuring so many of us think of and fear when the term is used, but just enough to help you with your present situation. You might want to consult a family or couples therapist, for example, or someone who is familiar with the problems faced by parents with sick children. With this kind of goal-oriented therapy, it's not at all uncommon for people to experience significant relief in a fairly brief amount of time.

Yet another cause of persistent anxiety may be a valiant effort to keep depression at bay. In fact, depression and anxiety are both signals that something is deeply wrong, but while anxiety is a heightened state of activity and awareness, depression produces a lessening of physical behavior. (Some anxiety is in fact an agitated depression, but only a professional can tell the difference.) There are people who use anxiety as a defense against depression, and people who use depression as a defense against anxiety.

Anger can also mask depression. Dr. Elinor Greenberg has observed that when men come to her for help with what they feel is an anger disorder, she frequently finds that they are in fact anxious or depressed—it's just that in our society anger is a more acceptable emotion for most men to express than anxiety or sadness. In women, it's frequently the opposite: many anxious or depressed women are frequently deeply angry women.

But understandably, many parents of allergic children confess to feelings of sadness and loss. You may feel sad, because you're grieving for the "perfect" child you feel you should have had, but didn't. You're sad, also, in advance, for that extra degree of difficulty your child will always have to deal with in his or her life. You may feel robbed of simple childhood joys—just stopping in at any cute ice cream shop and ordering a cone, let's say, without having to thoroughly question the server and ascertain if the ice cream is safe for your daughter to eat; or even something as simple as letting her eat the same birthday cake as everybody else. Or there may be a treasured family recipe for peanut butter cookies or lasagna that your son can't ever even taste.

On a deeper level, you may be feeling sad because having a child with serious food allergies means having to deal with the fact of your child's mortality on a daily basis. Indeed, when every trip to a restaurant or even a visit to a friend's house can feel like a walk through

Warning Signs of Depression

While sadness, feeling upset, and feeling blue are unavoidable and normal parts of life, depression is not. When you are depressed, you are not merely feeling tired, discouraged, and down. You are feeling that life holds little or no pleasure at all. (As one of Dr. Greenberg's patients eloquently put it, "Life has no sauce on it.") Just getting out of bed in the morning is a major undertaking. Accomplishing simple, day-to-day tasks can feel almost overwhelmingly difficult.

If you have experienced five or more of the following symptoms over the same two-week period, and if at least one of those symptoms includes either a continuously depressed mood or a loss of interest or pleasure in life, you may be suffering from depression.

1. A depressed mood most of the day, every day (whether sad or just curiously "empty"). You may be tearful, or you may just be unusually somber. If friends, coworkers, or family members have commented on your altered mood, even if you're not that acutely aware of it, it's significant. Some of us are skilled at hiding the truth from ourselves, but we can't always hide it from others.

2. A marked decrease of interest and pleasure in daily activities—a sort of "graying-down" effect—that lasts all day, every day.

3. A significant weight loss that was not achieved through diet, or a significant weight gain. People who are depressed frequently experience a change in appetite, with some eating far less and others eating a good deal more than usual.

4. A significant change in sleeping habits, either sleeping far more than usual (hypersomnia) or not being able to sleep much at all (insomnia).

5. Being either much more restless and agitated than usual, or slower and more lethargic.

6. Feelings of great fatigue and loss of energy nearly every day.

7. Feelings of worthlessness or excessive or inappropriate guilt.

8. A diminished ability to think or concentrate—a sense of walking around in a fog. Indecisiveness may be part of this. (If others have made comments to that effect lately, take heed; it may not always be as apparent to you as it is to others that you are significantly off your game.)

9. Recurrent thoughts of death or suicide without a specific plan or suicide attempt. You don't really, in your heart of hearts, *want* to die, but it represents an escape from the pain you're feeling.

Dysthymic Disorder

Depression's gentler sibling, dysthymic disorder is a graying-down state where getting out of bed isn't the issue, but not seeing much point to the whole exercise most definitely is. Some people seem to have been born dysthymic. They are the Eeyores of the world, slow to smile and even slower to be disappointed because they don't expect much from life anyway. Others experience dysthymia in reaction to an event or series of events: a divorce, perhaps, or the loss of a prized job, seeing the first signs of aging, or dealing with an unhappy family situation. Having to constantly monitor and deal with the demands of life with a seriously food-allergic child can tip people who are already prone to feeling a little blue over the edge into dysthymia or depression. Unlike people suffering from depression, dysthymic people aren't depressed all the time, day in and day out. But they feel down more often than not, most days of the week. If you have experienced two or more of the following symptoms for a significant period of time, you may be dysthymic and could benefit from help.

1. A change in your eating habits, either eating more or less than usual
2. Trouble falling asleep and/or staying asleep (insomnia) or a greatly increased need for sleep (hypersomnia)
3. Feeling tired and draggy a good deal of the time
4. Feelings of low self-esteem
5. A foggy state of mind, making it hard to focus or make decisions
6. Feelings of hopelessness and despair

enemy territory, a significant part of your mental energy goes to simply making sure that your child stays alive. You may even find yourself envisioning situations in which your child could die.

Sadness and grief go through predictable stages. Following the work of esteemed thanatologist Elisabeth Kübler-Ross, most psychologists today characterize those stages as: shock and denial, anger and rage, bargaining, disorganization and despair, and finally acceptance and hope. No matter what our psychological makeup, no matter what our reactions to painful experiences have been in the past, we all seem to follow the same trajectory through these different and difficult emotions. It's not always a straight path; we may reach a place of normalcy and peace, only to be devastated by having to deal with a serious reaction. And not surprisingly, some of those troublesome emotions may erupt when all is well; it's safer, after all, to give in to anger or despair when there is no clear and present danger demanding our immediate attention.

All of that is perfectly normal. No one dealing with a serious, day-to-day health issue can approach life with complete equanimity at all times. (How many of us can during the best of times, anyway?) The problems come when we get "stuck" at one stage or another for a prolonged period of time. We've all known or heard about people who can't seem to get past a certain level of coping no matter how long they've been dealing with a difficult situation: the angry, abrasive mother or father of an autistic child; the teary, fearful parents of a child with Down's syndrome or cerebral palsy; the anxious, high-strung mother who accompanies her child to school every day to make sure the child doesn't eat something/inhale something/react emotionally to something in a way that would require attention. It's a painful way to live, both for the affected parents as well as the child and other family members.

When someone is stuck in an emotional rut like this for a considerable length of time, feeling very bad and finding the tasks of everyday life to be much harder than they used to be, professionals call it an adjustment disorder. I've personally known several mothers of highly food-allergic children who fall into this category, and my heart goes out to them. They are intelligent, attractive, loving women who have experienced success in their careers and their relationships—winners by any standards. But their lives are ruled by their child's food allergy. Their anxiety about their child and sense of being overwhelmed spills over into everything they do, muddying even what should be easy, happy, relaxing times.

The common thread that runs through all of these disorders is a loss of that sense of rightness with the world that makes us able to face each day with some measure of grace. And the irony is, of course, that in no situation do we need that grace more than when we are dealing with a complex, sometimes scary issue that affects our children's very lives.

If you feel that you're having a difficult time coping with your child's food allergy, or if you have restricted your life in major ways as a result, it doesn't have to stay that way. You can get help and feel better rather quickly. Do it for yourself. Your whole family will benefit.

25

BROADENING OUR EMOTIONAL RANGE

Remember back in school when you learned that we humans use only about 1 percent of our brainpower for our day-to-day lives? As a follow-up, some teachers would also intone that *even Albert Einstein* used only about 2 to 3 percent of *his* brainpower every day. What an astonishing idea it was at the time! To think that we all have so much unused potential just sitting there waiting for us to use!

So it won't surprise you to learn that we all also have a much wider emotional range than we normally use. The bad news is, most of us are stuck in a pretty narrow band of the emotional spectrum. The good news is, our capacity to feel and behave in a variety of ways is what makes change possible.

Why *don't* we explore more aspects of our range? As with most issues relating to humans, it all boils down to comfort. When we find something that feels right, we stick with it. So even if being defensive, let's say, is creating a problem in our relationships, we may still feel more comfortable with our defense mechanisms than we would feel being open to criticism. Just the thought of being that vulnerable can make us feel terribly anxious. And since avoiding anxiety is a major motivator, we shut down.

Luckily, most of us lead full enough lives so that we are occasionally forced to behave in ways that stretch our comfort zone. While the defensive person may get away with crossing her arms and assuming a stony glare when criticized at home, that kind of behavior won't fly at the office. If one wants to be thought of as a team player, one has to at least *act* open to suggestions and be pleasant about receiving comments that may indicate room for improvement. Similarly, a tense, controlling person who can make the family feel as if they are walking on eggshells will generally make every effort not to openly berate his child or spouse in public. Both types have demonstrated that they are perfectly capable of acting differently. They just need to broaden the arena for that behavior, and practice it often enough so that the new way starts to feel as comfortable as the old way. If you've done it once, you can do it again.

There are many, many ways in which we can broaden our range. We can learn from our partner, from our friends, from family members, from role models, even from books. The only equipment we need is a willingness to try something new and the sense that every moment of our lives presents the opportunity for a fresh beginning.

Elinor Greenberg's favorite anecdote on this topic concerns an interview with the peerless Rudolf Nureyev. He was asked, "Mr. Nureyev, there are so many excellent male dancers. Why are *you* the *great* one?" Nureyev responded, "Other dancers practice what they do easily and well. *I* practice what I *don't* do so well!"

The chapter that follows describes coping styles and personality types that are recognizable to all of us. And virtually all of us will be able to quickly identify what camp we fall into. But remember, that's just a starting point—a default mode, if you will. Reading the descriptions, you may start getting a sense of what parts of your range you're relying on too much, and what parts you're neglecting. Although your core temperament and coping style may remain unchanged, it's helpful to learn that you can borrow strengths from other ways of behaving. Sometimes a controller just has to let it go; sometimes an avoider has to get down to brass tacks. But how? Look around you: there are plenty of teachers out there. We are all so much more—and capable of being so much more—than a thumbnail sketch of our personality types.

26

EMOTIONAL LEADERS AND TASK LEADERS

By the time we become parents, we've already developed our own ways of dealing with the world. And despite any efforts on our own or others' behalf, there's no real benefit to be had from trying to change the way we are—sunny or moody, low-key or intense—so long as we're fairly happy and functioning well. In fact, evidence suggests that temperament is inborn, with some variation for how we are raised.

Chances are, we've consciously or unconsciously chosen our partner based on how well our temperaments complement each other. We look for someone to give us balance and make us whole. Relatively early on in the relationship, we assign ourselves our roles. Someone is usually the "feeler," and someone is usually the "doer." Someone is the voice of reason, while the other roots for impulse. Someone has a greater affinity for maintaining family and social ties, while the other is more comfortable tending to the mechanics of running a home: budgeting the household expenses and paying the bills; keeping the house and car in reasonable repair; planning vacations; and the like.

In other words, someone is better suited to be the family's Emotional Leader, while the other makes a fine Task Leader, regardless of how you and your partner have actually apportioned your responsibilities.

The Emotional Leader knows how to keep everyone's morale up, creates a safe environment for expressing feelings, cushions the bad times, and celebrates the good. A gifted Emotional Leader keeps a family feeling cherished, connected, and proud of the connection. Bear in mind, however, that because Emotional Leaders think that tasks are less important than relationships and keeping everyone happy, they may not be as careful as they should be with details. Emotional Leaders are also not particularly good at making decisions, although they can carry out tasks once the decision has been made. And when it comes to matters of safety, Emotional Leaders may put psychological well-being over physical health. Some Emotional Leaders find it downright impossible to deny their child a few bites of a favorite food on special occasions, or will let their child eat an attractive treat without reading the ingredients, even if doing so puts the youngster at risk.

The Task Leader tends to the details: he or she is the one who gets things done and keeps the wheels of progress moving. A good Task Leader weaves a seamless fabric of well-being—the silver shines, everyone's hair is regularly cut, the car is in good repair, and the family's money is well-managed—which can be its own form of tender loving care. However, Task Leaders find it alien to address emotional issues. It's not in their makeup to notice that morale is sinking and family members are feeling depressed, just so long as ingredients labels are being read and the allergic child is safe. Task Leaders are interested in results; there is simply no such thing as an "A for Effort" in their book if you've missed some small detail along the way.

Both forms of leadership are vital for a healthy family to flourish. Appealing as it seems, you can't romp with the kids all day and have intense conversations all night while the bills go unpaid, the pipes burst, and no one ever makes it to the dentist. On the other hand, two people who are completely absorbed by the minutiae of daily existence probably aren't going to be able to create a very warm and satisfying home life.

Balance is the key. But, of course, perfect balance rarely happens.

Some families are obviously ruled by emotion, jumping into the car and driving off on great adventures at a moment's notice. Others raise their children in neat-as-a-pin homes where well-oiled routines are the order of the day. Both ends of the spectrum are perfectly wonderful ways to live, so long as everyone's needs for love and order are being met most of the time.

Allergies are the kink in the hose. A recent study titled "Impact of Food Allergy on Quality of Life" surveyed 400 families of food-allergic children. The results were presented at the annual meeting of the American Academy of Allergy and Immunology in spring 2000 and were reported in *Food Allergy News*. In brief, the findings were that childhood food allergy has a significant impact on emotional distress in parents.

Suddenly, the role of Task Leader is elevated to a position with life-or-death responsibility. Previously, if the bills got paid a few days late one month, or if the kids were a few weeks late for their yearly checkups, or if the checkbook didn't balance perfectly, nothing of earth-shattering significance would happen. But once a child is discovered to have food allergies, details are the essence of life itself. If a food label is improperly read (or not read at all), if sandwiches are put in the wrong lunch boxes, even if a waitress is not thoroughly quizzed on each and every ingredient of a meal, the consequences can be devastating.

What's more, the job is continuous, from the moment the child wakes up until bedtime. There is never any closure; never any sense of a task well done and complete. The neatly folded stack of laundry, still warm from the dryer, will, of course, turn into dirty clothes that just need washing again. But for a week, everyone will have clean clothes to wear, and laundry does not have to be uppermost in your mind. Food allergies must be uppermost in your mind many times a day, every single day of your life.

The Task Leader, who is not particularly comfortable with displays of emotion, is suddenly stuck with a job that is an emotional minefield. There is simply no breathing room for mistakes. Each and every last detail, every single time, must be meticulously examined and reexamined. If an accident happens, whether or not it was your fault, you are the one who will bear the brunt of the blame.

The ante is raised for the Emotional Leader as well. Now, instead of cheering your spouse on at work, having heart-to-hearts with older children, and just plain being the one everyone goes to for a smile, some advice, and encouragement, you are rallying the troops in an all-out war. Keeping everyone feeling good and cared for is a big job under any circumstances. But now you are the one called upon to keep a positive attitude, a cool head, and reassure everyone that everything will be all right, despite the fact that you may feel like doing nothing more than locking yourself in the bathroom.

Food allergies have a tendency to put everything under a microscope. The spouse who may have once seemed to be a paragon of trustworthiness and efficiency may turn out to be someone who was good about most details, but not a real stickler for accuracy. The spouse who was universally acknowledged to be the heart and soul of the family may in fact have been riding an emotional high—happy marriage, healthy children. When the chips are down, he or she may not be able to sustain that feel-good buzz.

Another common scenario, no less difficult to handle, is when it's necessary to reverse roles or take on both roles for the sake of the child. It can be very hard for a family when the person who has been comfortable being the Emotional Leader is suddenly handed a million details on a plate, or when the Task Leader has to assume the responsibility of keeping everyone's spirits up, because no one else in the family can keep cool in a crisis.

That's the bad news, and it can hurt in the beginning. Suddenly, someone you've always counted on to make you feel better, no matter what the circumstance may be, is having a hard enough time just getting through the day. Someone who has always been so gifted at juggling a myriad of tasks may be feeling overwhelmed just going to the grocery store. Someone who has never felt comfortable in certain situations—sticking out in a crowd, for example, or calling attention to a personal need—not only has to handle them every day but has to handle them with confidence and extreme competence.

Siblings Need Extra Care Too!

If your food-allergic child has a sibling or siblings without food allergies, don't assume that they are getting off easy. Yes, they are free
from the precautions and special arrangements that are a fact of life for
food-allergic children, but they are not immune to the stress of living
with an ever-present awareness of serious health issues. In fact, far
from feeling blessed to be free of allergies, many siblings express
resentment at all the attention and specially prepared foods the allergic
child receives. Some siblings will become overly concerned about the
food-allergic child, while others may act as though the thought never
crosses their minds. Understand that no matter what their actions are,
they are picking up both the spoken and unspoken emotions in the
house.

Feeling that we have received adequate attention as children allows
us to feel worthy of attention as adults. But as all parents quickly learn,
each child has his or her own definition of what adequate attention
means. One child will be happy with a book and special song at bedtime, while for another nothing less than attending every Little League
practice and game will do. Although good parents are always careful to
give each child special attention, the food-allergic child is virtually guaranteed his or her share. It's doubly important to attend to the needs of
our "easy" children.

Regardless of your family's style in the past, whether seat-of-the-
pants or spit-and-polish, you must now find a way to incorporate elements of both emotional leadership and task leadership into your
daily lives. If you stick to the nitty-gritty, emphasizing just task leadership, morale will go down. If you only have emotional leadership,
you're putting your child at risk.

And as if the two of you weren't enough to deal with, you also
have to recognize and be responsive to your child's own style. An
emotional child will need a different kind of parenting and guidance
than a task-oriented child.

The good news is that you can do this. You can do it *well*. All you
need is a commitment to your child's well-being, and a plan.

Be realistic. Sit down together one night, just the two of you, and decide between yourselves which of you is more comfortable handling the details and which one is better with emotions. If both of you are detail people, or if both of you are emotional people, that's all right too. Nobody is completely and fully one way or the other. And two heads are always better than one. Delegation is the key.

Together, make a list of things that need to be done in order to keep your child safe and your family happy. The list may look something like this:

1. Identify the unsafe foods in your house: everything from the jar of peanut butter to the egg-containing cake mix and whatever falls in between. (You'll have to read every label, so this may take a while.)

2. Decide what foods to throw away, what foods to give away, and which, if any, should be carefully labeled and kept out of your child's reach.

3. Choose a person to be in charge of reading labels and grocery shopping.

4. Choose a person to be in charge of cooking and preparing lunches for the allergic child. This includes researching and adapting recipes.

5. Designate someone as the "point person" to contact in case of emergencies.

6. Designate someone as the chief communicator to schools, day care, et cetera.

7. Choose a person to be in charge of medications. (This should be someone who is not only comfortable dealing with the doctor and the pharmacist, but also comfortable giving the medicine to the child.)

8. Make a plan for keeping the food-allergic child on a normal track. (What can be done to keep the child feeling safe but still "like other kids"?)

9. Make a plan for the nonallergic siblings, if any. (How can they contribute to the food-allergic child's safety without feeling as if they're having to give up too much? What special treats might they be missing out on that can be made up for in some way?)

Although this is a very basic list, it represents a lot of work. Even enthusiastic, well-balanced couples may find it daunting. In my experience, it can be very helpful to bring in a third party—a grandparent, a dear old friend, even a professional counselor—to help ease the burden.

Third parties are particularly useful in situations when the parents' style differs markedly from the child's. A task-oriented boy, for instance, may not feel quite secure despite the obvious efforts his emotional parents are making to keep him away from allergenic foods. He may need something more concrete: a laminated index card in his backpack with emergency instructions, for example, and a grown-up to talk to on a weekly basis about details and backup plans. An emotional boy being reared by task-oriented parents may feel a lack as well. His well-meaning parents may be patting themselves on the back for their level of organization and carefully constructed plans, when what he really needs is to be able to talk about his feelings and receive lots of extra love and reassurance.

You, better than anyone, know your child. You also know your limitations. If you cannot be as helpful to your child as you'd like to be, by all means bring in someone who can. It'll save wear and tear on *all* your relationships.

Just as we tend to be either Emotional Leaders or Task Leaders in our families, we tend to fall into one of two camps when it comes to managing anxiety: Controllers and Avoiders. Controllers make themselves feel better in difficult situations by taking charge. Avoiders make themselves feel better by deflecting attention away from the difficult situation, either telling themselves that things are not as bad as they seem, or fixating on something else.

And just as we tend to view the world in emotional or practical terms throughout life, our coping styles stay consistent as well. If in the past we've always managed to allay anxiety by playing the situation down, we'll want to do that with this new anxiety-provoking situation, our food-allergic child. If we've always handled worry by taking the bull by the horns, we'll feel most comfortable doing that now, too. As complex as we humans are, we are creatures of habit.

Those of you who are married to controllers may feel varying degrees of exasperation due to your spouses' needs to express an opinion about every detail of your lives together, and utter certainty that their way is always the right way. It may not hurt to bear in mind that you probably married this person because you wanted someone else to be in charge. And for better or for worse, that's what you got. If you choose to have a negative view of your mate, you can point to his or her bossiness, fussiness, and presumptions of being right all the time. If you choose to look on the positive side, however, you will probably find that you're married to someone who is comfortable with responsibility, can be counted on to make decisions, will keep the food-allergic child safe, and is always giving you input about issues that affect your lives together.

Avoiders, on the other hand, are people who manage anxiety by distracting themselves from the problem. They don't want any more information than is absolutely necessary—and even that small amount can seem too much to deal with. Some of them are carefree and starry-eyed; others are frightened and unsure. On the positive side, the avoiders in our lives can bring to the table a certain carefree, blithe spirit that lifts the moods of those around them—a mental vacation of sorts from the anxiety and worry that can all too easily infiltrate families of food-allergic children. Avoiders' refusal to let fear rule their life can be very freeing for their children and their partners. On the down side, avoiders can have difficulty facing facts and accepting that just wishing and acting as if their children have no restrictions doesn't make it so. It's perfectly wonderful to make positive assumptions about the world being a safe and good place, *once you've done your homework* and taken the steps necessary to ensure that it is.

If you are an avoider, it might not be a bad idea to carry a written emergency action plan with you whenever you are the sole caregiver for your child, and refer to it at the first sign of trouble. Make a pact with yourself that you will follow the instructions to the letter, *even if you feel they are too stringent,* and not give in to your natural tendency to brush all worries aside. Understand that your attachment to a carefree attitude could put your child in danger. And remember, it's not necessary or even desirable for you to change your overall outlook on life. You just have to make some adjustments in this one particular area.

If you are married to an avoider, you probably feel equal parts admiration and exasperation for this person's "don't worry, be happy" take on life. But when your child's health is on the line, the exasperation—plus generous doses of insecurity and fear—can rule. Your biggest task will be to help your partner acknowledge that there is a serious issue of ongoing concern in your lives and actively deal with that issue. Remember, life with an avoider can be fun and romantic—an avoider is the last person who will point out the bad and the ugly. So get your ducks in a row, then relax and enjoy the ride.

Unfortunately, some people who choose avoidance as their anxiety-management strategy of choice become blamers. Blamers either shift their anxiety to someone else or, as self-blamers, shift their anxiety inward.

Those who blame others do so because it is too deeply painful for them to contain guilt, fear, or other negative emotions within themselves. The result is that blamers yell and criticize, bluster and berate. And it's not always loud and messy. Blamers can speak softly and in a "reasonable" tone of voice, but the message is the same.

Self-blamers turn their guilt and anger inward: "If only I hadn't taken that medicine while I was pregnant," or "If only I hadn't introduced him to cow's milk so early," or "I know it's my fault—I had terrible eczema when I was a child." Self-blamers feel tremendous guilt.

Yet a third kind of dynamic can spring up when both partners decide that the two of them are perfect—it's the rest of the world that is to blame when something goes wrong. For example, if a child who is highly allergic to dairy is mistakenly allowed to eat a scoop of sherbet (which often looks like pure fruit but usually contains at least some milk) and the child experiences a reaction, both parents might agree that sherbet really ought not to contain milk in the first place and what was the manufacturer thinking by putting it in?

In many ways, growing up in this kind of environment presents the most danger to a food-allergic child. Without the benefit of at

least one parent who is willing to accept blame and the sense of control that blame implies, the child can feel at the mercy of a capricious world. What's more, because neither parent is willing to accept responsibility for his or her actions, the child will not learn to take the precautions necessary to stay safe. Blaming others may salve egos and explain away weaknesses when jobs fall through or deadlines aren't met, but when a child's health is on the line someone has to step up to bat.

Understanding where we are coming from gives us some perspective on our foibles, which in turn lets us compensate for them if we choose. Understanding where our partner is coming from allows us to predict with some accuracy how he or she will react in a given situation, and how we might be able to help. A healthy acceptance of our own and our partner's shortcomings—along with a reasonable plan to work around them—is one of the best things we can do not just for our food-allergic child but for all of our children.

27

FORGIVENESS

There may exist a child who once suffered a serious allergic reaction and never—whether through extraordinary vigilance, dumb luck, or a combination of the two—came into contact with that allergen again. It's possible. But I doubt it.

Most of us are both blessed and cursed to be living here in the real world, with all of its wonder and imperfections. We do not and cannot have complete control of our child's environment at all times. And while we should certainly not shrug our shoulders and accept an accident every few months or even once a year, many families' experience seems to suggest that an accidental exposure every few years may be part of the cost of doing business.

This is not to say that any accident—even the first in ten years—should be taken lightly. Depending on the severity of your child's allergy, an accident may be life threatening and traumatic for all involved. But we should all be aware that accidents can happen in even the most careful households: foods can be mislabeled; someone can forget to read an ingredients list because the child has been eating that food for years; or some form of cross-contamination can occur. We desperately don't want it to happen, but it does. That's why we always, always need to be prepared.

Of course, being prepared medically and being prepared emotionally are two entirely different things. As far as I know, no one has yet developed the parent's version of the EpiPen: after injecting your child with epinephrine, you inject *yourself* with a drug that ensures calm, equanimity, and a rational frame of mind. But we all could use it, for our entire family's sake.

Sorting out your feelings after your child has had an allergic reaction is a complex task. If you are the person who is responsible for the accident, or if you were the child's caregiver when the accident occurred, it can be devastating regardless of the circumstances. But you need to get through it and move on, as much for your child's sake as for your own.

- If you did something *right,* try to focus on that. Perhaps you *were* a bit too casual about letting your child eat a particular food. But once you saw the reaction beginning, you immediately began putting your emergency action plan into effect. You had all your medications on hand. You got your child to the E.R. And as a result, your child suffered as little as possible. He or she also learned that you can be counted on in a crisis.

- If you had a premonition that you dismissed—perhaps the packaged cookies, though labeled the same, looked different than you remembered; or you didn't feel completely confident in a particular waiter's ability to convey your request to the chef—forgive yourself for being trusting. It's better in the long run to be trusting than relentlessly paranoid. Now congratulate yourself for picking up on subtle cues that something was wrong. You've learned that you have good intuition. Next time, you will heed it.

- If the accident was completely unavoidable—mislabeled food, misinformed kitchen staff, or, as in my friend Ellyn's case, your child running ahead of you in a park and picking a peanut shell up off the ground—understand that even though *you* may have been the one to offer your child the food, order your child's meal in the restaurant, or take your child on the outing, *the accident was not your fault.* You cannot control the world. If you find that you can't help playing the what-if game ("what if I hadn't bought him that cereal, what if I hadn't let him have that hot dog"), sternly remind yourself that beating yourself up about issues out of your control is just another form of narcissism—and not even the fun kind, at that.

• If an accident caught you unprepared—no medication, no action plan—yet you managed to get your child help in a timely manner and he or she suffered no long-term consequences, you should certainly give yourself a good talking-to. You've seen the error of your ways; now change them. Your process of forgiveness can begin with gratitude for your child's life, a vow to never get caught short again, and a commitment to keeping that vow by immediately putting safeguards in place. Try to see the experience as a blessing in disguise: as a wake-up call, not a tragedy. Under different circumstances, the outcome may have been different. This time you got lucky. Take a deep breath, pack a meds bag, and move on.

We all have the potential to make mistakes. Even Dr. Sampson, one of the world's leading authorities on food allergy, once offered a bite of a mayonnaise-slathered sandwich to his egg-allergic daughter. (And yes, she had a reaction.)

If someone else was responsible for your child when the accident occurred, the issue of blame becomes even more complex. You may find yourself immensely angry at that person; blaming that person *and* yourself (because we parents have a highly refined sense of guilt when it comes to our children); or even blaming just yourself if you're predisposed to do it. ("I should have seen that situation coming and blocked it at the pass.")

If your spouse was the transgressor, first ask yourself if that makes it easier or harder for you to accept. Personally, I would rather my husband make the mistake than me, but not everyone feels that way. I have an easier time forgiving others than I do forgiving myself. No matter how your spouse is acting, it's safe to assume that he or she feels awful about what happened. Women, realize that men will sometimes try to play a situation down in order to calm *themselves* down. Inside they may be as deeply shaken as you, or even more shaken. If you start accusing them of not caring, they'll only withdraw more. Men, realize that women may need to obsess a little about what happened, retelling the story over and over again. Jumping in to describe what they could have done or how you would have handled it isn't very helpful at this point. Right now, she just needs your empathy.

If the accident occurred at day care, school, or camp, remember that you need to have an ongoing relationship with the people who work there. Try to find out what went wrong and what all of you, as a team, can do to prevent it from happening again. Blame, unless the situation was egregiously careless—a camp counselor handing out peanut butter cookies to all of the campers including your child, let's say—is simply beside the point. (And even in that situation, you would probably get better results by acknowledging that since food allergies can be hard to keep in mind at all times, your child should always bring a snack from home and never eat what the camp provides.) Give the people in charge the opportunity to tell their side of the story: you may learn something that will prove useful in the future. Ask them to present you with a plan to avoid future accidents. Remember, it could have been you. If you are going to keep your child in this particular day care, school, or camp situation, he or she must feel safe. Your forgiveness and trust are key elements in that equation.

Regardless of how or where the accident occurred, you and your spouse are going to have to sit down and have a heart-to-heart about it. Share your fears. Obviously, both of you have thought about what you would do and how you would feel if an accident happened. If you have always been afraid that you were going to be the one to make the mistake, and instead it was your spouse, share that with him or her. It should help take the pressure off a little. Share a cry or even a rueful laugh if you can summon it (let's face it, some allergic situations can border on the absurd), but understand that there is a price to pay for anger. It can ruin your relationship and your family. Sharing information brings people closer together; anger and blame drive them apart.

If your spouse was "on duty" when the accident occurred, ask yourself how you would want to be treated if it happened on your watch. How would your child want you to treat each other—and what is best for your child? Finally, what can the two of you learn from this? You may need to review your system and close a few loopholes, or you may need to come to terms with the fact that some accidents just seem to fall under the "act of God" proviso.

There is one situation, however, in which anger is not only justified but necessary: when someone who should know better is wantonly careless. Forgiveness is not the same as condoning or even tolerating unacceptable behavior. I know of at least one instance where a father allowed a child to eat a food that was known to be dangerous—cheese on a cheeseburger—because "all the other kids were having one." The little boy had an immediate, severe reaction and needed to be taken to the E.R. Needless to say, the mother was incredulous that her husband would actually allow such a thing to happen—and was absolutely furious about it. I don't think any of us would blame her.

When someone deliberately disregards your instructions concerning what your child can and cannot eat, whether or not a serious reaction follows, you are in a hostile situation. If the person is your child's teacher, you need to request a different teacher or change schools. If the person is a caregiver, you need to find another one. The point is that some people will find it nearly impossible to comply with your requests, for a variety of reasons. Some cannot tolerate the idea of "being told what to do." Others may have feelings about what a child needs to eat (milk and eggs, for example) that are so strong and deep-seated that they simply cannot grasp how deadly those foods can be. Still others may harbor anger that manifests itself in passive-aggressive ways. ("Oh, I know you said no milk for Dana, but who can eat a baked potato without butter?") When it comes right down to it, these situations are the easy ones.

It gets tricky when the people who are the greatest threat to your child—the grandfather who offers to buy your peanut-allergic child a nice big bag of peanuts at the ball game, the aunt who welcomes you to her home with great platters of peanut fudge and peanut butter cookies, the husband who can't say no at McDonald's—are the very people you love the most. You can't fire them. You can't replace them. And even if you and your husband divorced, he would probably get at least partial custody of your child. What do you do?

Clearly, each person presents a unique set of challenges. What drives the message home for Grandpa may simply alienate your aunt. And assuming you don't live in an extended-family situation, you probably do have a little time to think about what you're going to do. But because a parent is a child's primary caregiver, and the relationship between husband and wife is central to a child's sense of security, you need to get any unresolved issues relating to the child's allergies resolved immediately.

It's possible that your husband was so shaken by the reaction experience that he can be counted on to be the soul of discretion from here on in. Then again, maybe not. He may figure that since the child weathered that particular storm, other accidents will have a similar outcome. (Unfortunately, they may not—but it may be hard to convince him of that.) How you proceed depends on where he stands.

If your husband seems anxious and repentant, now is your moment. In as friendly, reassuring, and nonjudgmental a way as possible, make sure he knows what he needs to know (perhaps you'll want to jot down the "how to read an ingredients label" information from this book, or order some wallet cards from the Food Allergy Network) and has access to the action plan and meds he'll need in order to handle any unforeseen reactions in the future. Right now, with the memory of the accident fresh in his mind, is when he is most receptive to the idea of changing his behavior.

If your husband truly doesn't seem that ruffled by the experience—or even takes pride in how he pulled off the save—and you find the near-miss intolerable, the two of you clearly have a lot to work on. But remember that forgiveness doesn't necessarily begin and end with an actual incident. Many of us are in situations where one spouse is consistently more cautious and conservative than the other in terms of handling a child's food allergy. Over time, we can begin to harbor resentments almost unawares. Soon resentments build up, and energy that could have gone into replenishing our relationships drains out of them instead.

Forgiveness is ultimately a highly practical act because it is both healing and freeing. But it cannot always be rushed. It may take a while before you can forgive your partner or your partner can forgive you for an incident involving your child's well-being. But when the anger is spent, forgiveness is the only way to move on—perhaps even to a deeper relationship that acknowledges fragility and the possibility of loss while embracing growth.

28

A ROUNDTABLE DISCUSSION ON RAISING A CHILD WITH FOOD ALLERGIES

If it's one thing I've learned about raising a child with food allergies, it's that different parents have very different experiences. And everyone has something valuable to teach about navigating this often-tricky terrain, even if it's just a recounting of the one mistake he or she will never make again. To this end, I invited four mothers who have each been dealing with food allergies for at least five years to join me in a roundtable discussion on the issue. Our purpose was twofold: to speak freely on the special challenges we have encountered in raising our children, so that all of you in the same situation know that you're not alone; and to offer support to all who may be new to the world of food allergies or who have not yet encountered certain situations (sending your child off to school, dealing with uncooperative teachers, bringing a child to the E.R.) where guidance would be most helpful.

I had prepared a list of questions to keep us on track, but I was as interested in the digressions as I was in sticking to the agenda. As we all know, the truth comes out when it will.

The moms in this discussion are: Bridget, mother of three, all with food allergies; Stacy, mother of two, one with food allergies; Kate, mother of four, one with food allergies; and Helen, mother of four, all with food allergies. I am a mother of two, one with food allergies.

MARIANNE: Let's open this discussion by sharing how each of us found out about our children's food allergies, and take it from there.

BRIDGET: My first son was four months old when he had his first allergic reaction. I was feeding him peas and blueberries from baby food jars—he had his vegetable and his fruit; I thought I was doing a good job!—and he just transformed in front of my eyes. He swelled up so badly that his eyes almost shut. I grabbed him out of the chair, and we went straight to the doctor's office. Frankly, I don't even remember what they gave him, although I know it wasn't an EpiPen. I was in too much shock. That was the beginning of the learning curve for me, and in some ways it feels like we're still there.

STACY: When my son was four and a half, they were doing an arts and crafts project in nursery school, making bird feeders. You roll a pine cone in peanut butter and stick the birdseed on. The teacher called me and said, "You'd better come down here right away. Ben's face is so swollen that his eyes are closed, and we don't know what's wrong." When I got to the school, another teacher said, "Be sure to tell your doctor that he was working with peanut butter." That never would have occurred to me. Ben had never eaten peanut butter before—he just said he didn't like it. But when I went to the allergist, she said that the first thing she tests for is the food a mom says her child absolutely refuses to eat. It's a natural foreboding that children seem to feel. And sure enough, it was the peanut butter that did it.

BRIDGET: It's amazing how times have changed in the past eight years. There's so much more awareness now. When my oldest son was in school, there was a no-medication policy; the school could not give an EpiPen or even Benadryl to a child having an allergic reaction. I had to write all these letters to the school board explaining why the policy needed to be changed, and I even joined the board myself. Now most schools are very cooperative. The teachers are EpiPen trained. Some nursery schools are even nut-free.

KATE: My other two daughters always ate peanut butter and jelly sandwiches, but my daughter Elizabeth wouldn't—she said she didn't like it. Then, on Thanksgiving Day, she touched a peanut shell and she blew up; her tongue and her face were completely swollen. We took her to an allergist who did a CAP RAST blood test. When the results came back, the allergist told us to get an EpiPen and that Elizabeth had to stay away from even a trace of peanuts. We learned how careful we truly had to be when she was five: she was at someone's house, and a little baby who had just eaten peanut butter crackers came up to her and touched her on the face. Elizabeth immediately blew up again, and she remained swollen for three days, even on the Atarax the doctor prescribed.

HELEN: All of my children have had extremely sensitive skin and itchy, rashy eczema that can get to the point of being bloody. When my older son was just a newborn, I put him down in the crib so I could quickly go do something, and when I came back just a few minutes later he had traveled all the way to the other end. I thought, what a wonderfully strong and active baby! But it turns out he was so active because his skin was so itchy. When he was about three, our doctor suggested that we give him the tiniest taste of peanut butter. He liked it at first, then started crying and said he hated it. Within minutes his face was so swollen he was unrecognizable. Needless to say, that doctor doesn't recommend giving any possibly allergic child a taste of peanut butter anymore! When my daughter was sixteen months old, she ate some sesame noodles made with peanut butter and complained that her tongue was tingling. A few months later at our club, she ate a cookie made with nuts and immediately vomited, then developed hives on her face.

MARIANNE: How long would each of you say it took to make the adjustment to dealing with the fact that your child has a serious food allergy? And what would you say made it easier or harder to deal with?

BRIDGET: I think we're still adjusting to it now!

KATE: It's very scary. I think when I got that diagnosis—asthmatic, peanut allergy, chance of her having another anaphylactic reaction—I just wanted to put her in a bubble and not bring her anywhere.

STACY: I found out that my father was dying the day before Ben was diagnosed with his peanut allergy. So I had to give up responsibility for Ben very quickly in order to be with my dad, who needed me more. I had to teach people how to use an EpiPen and what Ben could eat. Going through it was awful and very emotional, but in the long run it probably helped me because I didn't have time to give in to that fear or keep him close to me. I was dropping him at friends' houses and saying, "I'll be back in five hours. This is what he can eat, and this is how to use an EpiPen." I couldn't really focus on it. I just had to do it and survive.

KATE: That sounds awful, but I think something like that would have helped me, too. For me, it was very hard to leave Elizabeth. I only trusted my mother and mother-in-law as baby-sitters. When she went to parties, I always stayed at the parties. For me, it was very scary.

BRIDGET: I feel that I've always taken a less cautious approach than many people. I didn't have the kids carry the EpiPens with them even though the doctor said I should, because I didn't want to burden them or make them feel different. Part of it was my own denial and even a little ignorance. When my middle child had his reaction, he was at family day care and the day care provider knew what was going on because my older son had been with her, too. She had given him bread from a health food store, and he began to have a reaction. She called me at work, and we agreed that she'd give him some Benadryl and call me back to let me know what was going on. She called back pretty quickly and said that he was in bad shape. His lip was so swollen it had split. At that point I called my husband, and we zoomed over to the pediatrician. When he was a baby, there were signs that he was allergic, but I just didn't catch it. In hindsight I think: how could I not have known? But [at the time] you're not looking for it.

STACY: Until you're living it, you just don't know it.

BRIDGET: That's right. Also, I'm definitely an "oh, you're all right" kind of mom, which doesn't always work. Sometimes they really are sick. But my husband is more the worrier.

HELEN: My biggest concern always is that my children enjoy their lives and feel that they can do anything. They have to take care of their bodies, but I don't want them ever to feel limited. I don't want them to be afraid of living!

BRIDGET: I think one thing that was especially hard for me was it just seemed improbable that all three of them would have to deal with this. The thing that's been most frustrating is their diets, because what they'll eat is so limited and so different that I end up being a short-order cook, and basically none of them eat well. I always took the approach that if they don't want to eat something, it's their bodies telling them not to—so don't push it. But now basically all my oldest eats is bread and milk, so clearly that approach isn't working. We're going to test them all again and see what's really going on.

HELEN: When in doubt, we just try to stick with very plain food: broiled chicken, vegetables, fruits they can have, that sort of thing. You can find that kind of food pretty much anywhere, although you have to be very specific about how plain it has to be. But we like our junk food too, and we've got plenty of the safe kinds at home at all times!

BRIDGET: One day at nursery school, the teachers gave my son a chocolate chip cookie from a bakery. When I came to pick him up, his lip was swollen, and playing the detective I began asking questions about what he ate, what was in it, all that. We located the package the cookie had come in, and I immediately saw how the contamination had occurred: his cookie had been packed in the same box as a bunch of peanut butter cookies. Of course you don't want to upset the kid and blow up at the teacher right then and there; you just try to deal. But by the time we got to the pediatrician, he had a full-blown reaction going. Then, a week later we thought he had a bladder infection because he kept urgently having to go to the bathroom every few minutes. It turns out it was a syndrome common in four- to five-year-olds that can be brought on by a fear that they are going to die. Luckily, it cleared up on its own in a few weeks.

MARIANNE: Actually, it might interest all of you to know that the Food Allergy Network just released a study monitoring the stress reported by families dealing with different chronic childhood illnesses, including food allergies, epilepsy, and asthma. The families dealing with the food allergies reported the highest levels of stress overall.

STACY: Isn't that interesting! But you know, it makes sense because our dangers are so often hidden.

KATE: That's true, and my husband hasn't always been on the ball about things. Once he took my daughter to a baseball game without her EpiPen. Peanuts everywhere! And sure enough, she started to get a reaction. Somehow they got hold of some Benadryl and she was OK, but that was very frustrating to me. He'd take all four girls out for ice cream, and I'd say, "Do you have the EpiPen?" and he'd say, "No. C'mon, Kate, you're overreacting." But then he saw her when she was all blown up for three days, and I think it sunk in how serious this was.

STACY: We keep an EpiPen thumbtacked to the entrance to the garage in a big red bag so my husband can't miss it—and even then, I still have to remind him.

KATE: The nice thing now is that my daughter is about to turn thirteen and she's totally responsible. She won't eat anything she's not completely sure about. She's kind of neurotic in a way—she remembers that bad reaction—but remembering it will protect her.

STACY: We have to walk such a fine line between instilling a healthy fear and keeping them happy, normal children.

KATE: The teenage years are scary in that the peer pressure starts kicking in. You have to start worrying about them going out with their friends.

MARIANNE: I even worry about things like kissing. If you're allergic to peanuts and you kiss or even hold hands with someone who's just eaten anything with peanuts in it, you're probably going to have a reaction.

BRIDGET: I give my husband the EpiPen bag when I'm going to be away for the day, but I have to admit that I'm not as good about it as I should be. Yes, it's always in the car, but I need to stay more on top of checking the expiration date, making sure it's not in the hot sun or in a cold car overnight—that sort of thing. We've also had episodes when we probably should have given my son an EpiPen and didn't—we chose to go to the doctor. I know in my heart I would do it if I really felt he absolutely had to have it right then, but I'd rather have the shot come from the doctor than me because there's such a fear there.

STACY: I had to give Ben an EpiPen once, which was a horrible experience but also a fabulous experience because it showed me that I could give him an EpiPen if I needed to, and it showed Ben that we could handle an allergic reaction. Our emergency plan works.

We were at a birthday party that was held in the morning, so I just brought a piece of cake for Ben. Then at 10:30 the mom brought out two platters of sandwiches, peanut butter and tuna fish. Ben wanted a tuna sandwich. So I got a fresh piece of bread, scooped the tuna off the bread it was on, put it on the new bread, and gave it to him. But they must have used the same knife for the tuna as they did for the peanut butter, because within minutes he said, "Mommy, my lips hurt." Then he said, "Mommy, my tongue hurts," and his whole face just started welting up. The difficult decision was the decision to use the EpiPen—even though it just took around a minute for me to reach it. But once I came to that decision, it was actually an easy thing to do. I said, "Ben, we need to use the EpiPen, and I need you to come sit down next to me." Then I had someone call 911 and someone call my husband to say that everything's fine but meet us at the hospital.

After I gave him the EpiPen, we went out front to wait for the ambulance. I didn't want all the emergency personnel swooping down on the birthday party. The ambulance pulled up right away. They were so kind. They hooked him up to the EKG—because of the epinephrine, his heart rate was really high, and that was scary to me—but they really tried to make it as good an experience as possible for him. They took him to the hospital, where he was observed for four hours and then placed on steroids for four days. As terrifying as it was, we got through it, and I will never forget that.

What's interesting to me is that when I gave him the sandwich, I had this feeling deep down inside that told me to watch him carefully—this might not be safe. It should have been a red flag. But I purposely ignored it. We were just six months into dealing with peanut allergy—six months of people telling me I was a little neurotic and I should just ease up a bit. So I said to myself, Stacy, if he wants tuna fish, let him have tuna fish.

I didn't look into my own heart. Now I know that he needs to be protected, and if I need to have stringent rules, that's the way it's going to be. And it's very important for him now, as he's growing older, to learn to take over some of that control. He's going to have to make the right decisions.

BRIDGET: I guess that's the one good thing about my kids not eating anything! I don't have to worry about what they're eating when they're out of the house. It's almost a nonissue.

KATE: It's the asthma that scares me. When Elizabeth has a reaction, there's just not the comfort level that we'll be able to easily take care of it. That's why she just can never have a reaction! We had one instance recently when Elizabeth really wanted a cookie that someone else had baked, and she was really giving me a hard time that she couldn't have it. I finally turned to her and said, "Elizabeth, do what you want to do. It's in your hands. I'm only your mother." Of course she got really mad at me—she said, "Mom, it's all your fault that I can't have it!"—but she didn't eat the cookie.

BRIDGET: I also think that when we were growing up, we didn't go out to dinner as much. You just didn't have the variety that we have now. You didn't have sushi in the grocery store! You had meat, potatoes, salad, and that was it, every night.

STACY: There are so many different types of ethnic foods that we're all exposed to now . . .

BRIDGET: . . . and we think that we're doing good by exposing our children to so much this and that.

KATE: But now I don't think that we are. I don't know about you, but I don't like going out to dinner with Elizabeth.

BRIDGET: It makes me very anxious.

STACY: We go out for Italian food or nothing. Occasionally Mexican. But luckily I only have to check for peanut. I will take Ben to a restaurant if there are no peanuts on the premises. If there are peanuts in the kitchen, we don't go. But I don't have to ask about walnuts or pine nuts or almonds, which I know are a problem for a lot of people.

BRIDGET: The other thing that makes me crazy is the kid shampoos. It seems that every kid shampoo has almonds or melon or something else that my kids have to stay away from.

MARIANNE: When Lucas was a toddler, one of the nurses in our pediatrician's office pointed out a brand of diaper rash ointment that had peanut oil in it. People just don't realize the huge ripple effect it has on your life when your child is so allergic to one food.

BRIDGET: Over spring break we took a vacation, and we had to fly. When the flight attendant came around with the peanuts, I took a bag for me. But then I called her aside and asked if she could log a comment that I was flying with three peanut-allergic kids, there are lots of kids with peanut allergy, and maybe it would be better if the airlines handed out pretzels instead.

STACY: They will, but you have to call them ahead of time. We always call the airlines a month before to have them put a no-peanuts request in the manifest. When we get to the airport, we check again. Then I always pre-board and check under the seats for peanuts the cleaning crew may have missed. I also wipe off the tray table. We actually had a wonderful experience with one airline that made an announcement before boarding that this was a nut-free flight, and asked passengers to refrain from bringing or eating peanut snacks on the plane. Then the pilot came out to meet Ben and told him that when he was little he had a food allergy, and he just wanted Ben to know that the airline is aware of allergies, and that Ben doesn't have to worry about the flight.

HELEN: My older daughter went to a birthday party once where the mom had baked this absolutely beautiful Barbie cake—completely decorated, outfit and all. But Alexandra couldn't eat it because we didn't know the exact ingredients, and even though she's usually very good about these things, she felt pretty sad. Well, two days later, when Alexandra had a play date over at the birthday girl's house, the mom brought out a cake that was identical to the one at the birthday party—this time made completely safe for my daughter. I was really pretty overwhelmed at that.

KATE: I think that food allergies are becoming more common now, and people are becoming more cooperative. I've had teachers who have really been sensitive and good about it. Last year, though, we did have an incident when a substitute teacher did a science experiment with legumes and brought in peanuts. That was a little bit scary, but I made a call to the school and thought it was settled. Then the substitute came back the next week and still had that bag of peanuts. At that point I got pretty angry and called the school superintendent. Since then, they have definitely changed their attitude and have really been more proactive and helpful in thinking of things that I don't even think of.

HELEN: Our most difficult situation so far was with my daughter's kindergarten teacher. She was very controlling, and she liked to use candy as manipulatives for learning. The year my daughter was in her class, I asked if we could use candy Alexandra could eat, like certain kinds of jelly beans and gummy bears, instead of candy that was known to have nuts or nut traces in it, but this teacher just wasn't going for it. Alexandra ended up using her special candy for manipulatives while the rest of the class used the other kind, and it was hard for her at times. It made me nervous, because if you have someone in charge of your child, you want them to be sincerely interested in their welfare—not just paying lip service to it. It's scary when you have authority figures who question just how genuine a food allergy is.

Of course, I know that food allergies can be really confusing for people who don't know a lot about them. For instance, I always try to pack my children a balanced meal for lunch, complete with fresh fruit. But during certain seasons, particularly spring, they experience oral allergy syndrome—an itchy mouth—when they eat fresh fruit. So sometimes it's OK for them to eat the fruit, and sometimes it isn't. I know that the teacher thinks I'm being wildly inconsistent and even contradictory, but that's just because she won't take the time to listen or learn about the allergy.

BRIDGET: I feel like there's always going to be something. If we use Skittles or jelly beans, then there are going to be kids who are allergic to the red dye. I've been more interested in teaching my kids that they have to deal with their allergies. By always teaching them that they can avoid the bad situations, it doesn't train them—and I think they have to be trained. Even when my oldest was four, he knew what he couldn't have. I think you can get into this thing when you make everybody avoid the allergen, and suddenly the responsibility is on everyone but the children. They need to go through that hurt of not being able to have what everyone else is having in order to learn.

STACY: I must admit, I buy a lot of chewy junk food so that when Ben comes home with something he can't eat, he just gives it to me and he gets his gummy worms or whatever he likes, and for now that's working—just trading things.

MARIANNE: What was the most helpful thing for all of you in dealing with your child's food allergy?

STACY: I would say number one was the Food Allergy Network.

KATE: Without a doubt.

STACY: I also have a handful of friends who have embraced this issue so phenomenally well. They have kept their houses virtually peanut-free just so we can eat at their homes. My closest friend keeps her peanut butter in a jar wrapped in a plastic baggie in her refrigerator. She has so educated herself on the topic that I can leave Ben at her house without even saying a word. I just hand her the EpiPen and walk out.

MARIANNE: Unfortunately, it can sometimes go the other way, too. We have found that even the people closest to us, who truly have our best interests at heart, can make big mistakes. When Lucas was extremely allergic to milk, we had a lot of people pour him glasses of milk by mistake. I usually caught it in time, but one time he took a sip, said "Mommy, this tastes funny," and a few moments later he was breaking out in big, welting hives, and I was pouring a teaspoon of Benadryl down his throat.

BRIDGET: That's true. My mother-in-law just gave the kids big chocolate Easter bunnies, and on the back of all of them it says "traces of peanut." She was just thinking "chocolate," but you can't do that.

HELEN: My father, who knows so much about food allergies and loves my kids so much, once offered to buy my daughter peanuts when they were on an outing together. We've had similar situations with my sisters, too. Once when we were having a picnic, one of my sisters brought out ice cream cones with crushed peanuts on them for her kids, and plain ice cream cones for mine. She figured that would be OK. But I had to point out to her that crushed peanuts fall off the cone, plus I had a baby who would put anything he saw on the picnic blanket in his mouth. Then she got it, but it just hadn't occurred to her that there might be a problem.

BRIDGET: I don't leave my kids with family members because they just don't get it. Plus, we're dealing with so many environmental allergens too—they're allergic to cats and dogs—and my parents have a farm. So we'd go visit the farm, and we'd be right back at the pediatrician's office with swollen eyes and ear infections. The doctors finally said, "You really can't visit your family," which was awful. Think of it—the kids would have each had their own horse to ride, all these great animals around, but we just couldn't do it. We got so into frogs because they don't have fur!

MARIANNE: Bridget, what advice would you give parents who are just receiving a diagnosis of food allergy?

BRIDGET: Well, it's like anything else—it's the pendulum effect. You start off all worried, then you get less so. Maybe I'm at that stage right now, and I've got to come back to the middle a bit. It's all about finding what works for you and trying to stick with that.

KATE: I always find that in August and September when school starts is the worst time for me. My anxiety goes way up, and I am really stressed out. Even as Elizabeth is getting older, it's not getting any better.

BRIDGET: I feel like I always have to play the part of the nag, writing the letter to the teacher that sort of sticks it to her, basically saying, "If anything happens to my son, I'm holding you responsible."

STACY: I know. I always think, boy, this is not such a great way to get a start on the school year. Because whenever I'm talking to people who don't know Ben—new teachers, new counselors, waiters in restaurants—I always use the term *life threatening* to describe his allergy. When you say those words, they look at you differently.

KATE: They don't want to have to call 911 and wait for the ambulance.

STACY: That's right. I've been using the words *life threatening* since Ben was four and a half, when he didn't really understand the full impact of what I was saying. But now there's no doubt that he knows exactly what those words mean. And that has been very upsetting to me, that a child should know his life is in danger if he eats the wrong thing. That was a very sad realization.

MARIANNE: I never said to Lucas that he could actually die from eating peanuts. I would say, "You'll get very, very sick, and you'll have to have an EpiPen and go to the hospital." That was plenty of warning for him. But one of his teachers told the class that Lucas could die from peanuts, and he came home that day white as a sheet and asked if it was true. I had to tell him that it was, but that it was extremely unlikely because we are always so very careful about his food.

KATE: In their teen years, I think, when they want to start fooling around with things, you have to be really clear and strict about it. You have to tell them they could die.

STACY: You hate to do it, but you have to.

MARIANNE: If there was something that you could tell parents who have just received an allergy diagnosis for their child—that hard time when you first find out how much your life is going to have to change—what would you tell them?

KATE: I would tell them that right now it's going to seem overwhelming and that they can't do it, but there's a lot of support out there: there's the Food Allergy Network; there are people who have been through the same thing. It's definitely doable. You can have a healthy, happy, normal kid who lives to a ripe old age, and you've got to believe that and be positive about it.

HELEN: The most important thing is not to panic. You need to keep your child a balanced person who lives in the real world. We need to develop children who are secure. It's the child's emotional well-being that counts most of all.

STACY: I was so overwhelmed when I first found out about Ben's allergy. I needed to process all the information. I think it takes a good six months to figure it out. But once you do and you set up a life, it's just like any other limitation. You learn to live with it. When I meet with a camp counselor or a teacher, the first thing I'm always sure to say is "Ben is a normal, healthy, fabulous, typical eight-year-old who happens to be allergic to peanuts." I really want to try to get people to look at that. He's a normal kid who just can't eat everything. And I think that's really the most important thing we're trying to instill in Ben and the people around him. There's so much worse out there.

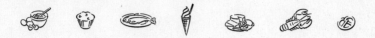

PART III

Itching, Sneezing, and Wheezing

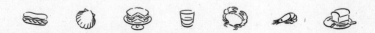

29

ASTHMA

As many as 50 percent of food-allergic children also have asthma or environmental allergies. No great surprise there; if you have a food allergy, you've already demonstrated that you have an immune system fully capable of mounting an allergic response. In fact, one of the major risk factors for developing a food allergy is having a close family member with *any* sort of allergy, from the exact same food allergy to hay fever to an allergy to mold, dust, or animal dander. Some food-allergic children actually suffer more from their asthma and environmental allergies than they do from the food allergy; others have only mild allergic symptoms or even none at all. If your child has food allergies but no asthma or environmental allergies, take heart: he or she might very well never develop them. The odds are in your favor. If, however, your child is already showing signs of asthma, environmental allergies, or both, you can take heart, too: treatments for asthma are better and easier than ever before, and keeping your home allergen-free is not at all difficult after the initial effort.

While asthma does not make all (or even most) children seriously ill, we'd be remiss not to take all of its symptoms seriously. Asthma is the leading cause of hospitalization in children. Learning your child's triggers and onset symptoms—and paying close attention to them—gives you the most control over your child's asthma and helps keep minor to moderate episodes from escalating into scary ones.

The main point to keep in mind is that, as with food allergies, the key to keeping your child healthy is plain and simple avoidance. If the asthma is triggered by animal dander, you'll almost certainly need to give up a family pet (sad and difficult as that is) and try to avoid visiting homes where pets live. If the asthma or rhinitis (nasal symptoms) is activated by dust mites, you'll need to keep your child's bedroom as stripped down as possible and see where you can make changes in the rest of the house. If mold and mildew are the problem, keeping your house dry is key. Grass and pollen allergies can be controlled indoors by keeping the windows closed during spring and fall months, running the air conditioner to cool things off when necessary. All of these (and more, in the sections to come) are simple, low-cost, practical measures that can make a world of difference to your child. The more you know, the better off your child will be. For once you discover which allergy or allergies are causing the problem, you can do something about it—sometimes immediately. Here's how.

WHAT IS ASTHMA?

Asthma is typically defined as a chronic disease of the airways. Technically, of course, that's an irrefutably accurate definition; asthma *is* chronic, meaning once you've got it, you can expect symptoms to come and go for years (because no one has yet found a magic bullet that will cure it). But personally, I have always hated that definition because it sounds so grim. For most of us, living with asthma means dealing with a child who is healthy at least as often as he or she is sick. (Although during the winter months it may not seem that way.) Some of us, unfortunately, will have a rather long siege ahead, during which time it will feel as though we're devoting an inordinate amount of energy to just keeping our child breathing. But whether serious or mild, once your child has been diagnosed with asthma, you do need to keep that fact in mind, even if you're one of the lucky ones whose child goes a year or more between episodes. An airway that has overreacted once will most likely overreact again at a later date.

Those of us who don't have asthma seldom have cause to think about our breathing. We breathe in; air flows easily into our lungs. We breathe out; air flows easily out. Aside from the occasional cough or congestion, breathing is just one of those things that we happily take for granted.

Not so for people with asthma. Children suffering with asthma have described their symptoms variously as "an elephant sitting on my chest," "a cough that goes all the way down to my stomach," "a ball of feathers stuck in my throat," and "I can't get the air out of my lungs"—all highlighting the difficulty of taking a normal breath. During an asthma episode (*attack*, a word often used to describe asthma, sounds scary in and of itself, and I avoid it at all costs), the airways inside your child's lungs react to an environmental or viral trigger by swelling, going into spasm, and becoming clogged with mucus. To see for yourself what an asthma episode feels like, take a

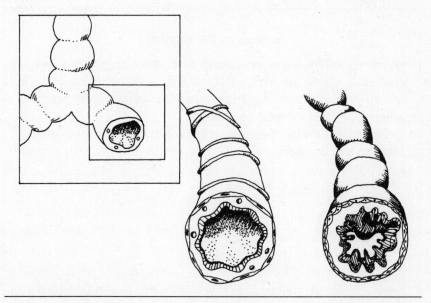

Healthy bronchial tubes (inset and drawing on left) are open and smooth. During an asthma flare (drawing on right) the muscles tighten and spasm, and the tubes become clogged with sticky mucus, making breathing difficult.

deep breath of air, hold it, then try to inhale again. Try to breathe in more air after that, and after that. In less than a minute, your chest will feel ready to explode. The problem for children with asthma is not inhaling; it's exhaling. Carbon dioxide has to go *out* so that good oxygen can come *in*.

Asthma is an *inflammatory* disease. The bronchial tubes of a person with asthma—even very mild asthma—are always a bit swollen, even when the person is showing no overt symptoms. That explains why your child may seem to develop breathing difficulties so rapidly. (In fact, the word *asthma* comes from an ancient Greek word meaning "panting.") The onset may *seem* like an acceleration from zero to sixty in just a few minutes, but in fact your child may already have been at thirty to forty for a few days, and was probably never much below fifteen or twenty. Much like children with extremely sensitive skin that flushes, breaks out, or chaps at the slightest change in soap or weather, the airways of children with asthma are always in a reactive state. All it takes is the right trigger to put them in reaction mode.

Asthma by the Numbers

Not only is asthma a time-consuming illness, it is a costly one as well. A child with asthma will likely make more trips to the doctor and will require more prescription medicine than a child who does not have asthma and is in otherwise good health.

Each year in the United States, asthmatic children from birth to their fifteenth birthday will:

1. Make 3,028,000 doctor visits
2. Go to the emergency room 570,000 times
3. Be hospitalized 164,000 times
4. Need 8.7 million prescriptions
5. Miss more than 10 million school days

Sources: (1 and 2) National Ambulatory Medical Care Survey, 1993–95; (3) National Hospital Discharge Survey, 1994; (4) National Medical Expenditure Survey, 1987; (5) *New York Times*.

Another kind of asthma is *exercise-induced asthma* (EIA). While many, if not most, children with allergic asthma will experience some asthma symptoms during intense exercise, children with true EIA will *only* experience their symptoms at those times. Often, a combination of high activity and cold, dry air seems to be the culprit. Happily, EIA is easily controlled and is seldom serious.

WHAT HAPPENS IN AN ASTHMA EPISODE

When a child with asthma is exposed to a trigger—cold air, a viral infection, an allergen—a chain reaction begins. The muscles around the airways go into spasm, causing the airway to tighten and narrow. Then the mucous membranes within the bronchial tubes go into overdrive, producing large amounts of mucus, which clog the airway even more. It's this combination of muscle spasm and increased mucus flow within the lungs that produces the wheeze, cough, and difficulty in breathing that are the hallmarks of an asthma episode.

CAUSES OF ASTHMA

In general, being born into an allergic family—no matter what the allergies are caused by—increases a child's risk of developing asthma at some point in his or her life. It is estimated that about one third of all children with asthma have a member of their immediate family with asthma, too. Seventy-five to 80 percent of children who have asthma have some sort of allergies as well.

Although infant eczema is not technically a predictor of whether a child will develop asthma, about half of all babies with moderate to severe eczema will experience asthma at some point. The most interesting correlation seems to be between egg allergy and asthma: 35 percent of all egg-allergic children go on to develop asthma.

Some food-allergic kids experience asthma symptoms only when they have accidentally ingested the wrong food. Others, who have environmental allergies as well, may also find it rough going at certain times of the year (spring's pollens and fall's molds in particular) or when they come into contact with indoor allergens such as dust mites (in carpeting, curtains, upholstered furniture, and stuffed animals, and on windowsills, blinds, and furniture), animal dander (from the furry family pet), feathers (in pillows, down comforters, upholstered furniture, down outerwear, or the family bird), and mildew (in bathrooms and anywhere damp).

Many children with asthma will experience symptoms when they have upper respiratory infections or any other illness, during vigorous activity, or upon exposure to cold air. Most children with asthma react to the vapors released by household cleansers, wet paint, new carpeting, or any other strong, irritating odor. If you have a gas oven, you should know that many children with asthma react strongly to the nitrogen oxide these ovens release. Some children with severe tree pollen allergies may find that their symptoms are marked during the spring, then come back during the holiday season, when evergreens with their molds and resins festoon homes, restaurants, and stores.

Research indicates that children who develop respiratory infections caused by *Chlamydia pneumoniae*, *Mycoplasma pneumoniae*, adenovirus, or respiratory syncytial virus (RSV) are at increased risk for developing asthma. Interestingly enough, however, being exposed to other sorts of infections may actually *protect* children against developing asthma, by stimulating their immune systems. Some researchers have found that children living in large families—who are naturally exposed to a wider variety of infectious organisms—are less likely to develop asthma than children from small families. Like food allergies, asthma is an example of how our sanitized world creates new health problems as it eliminates others.

Children who live in buildings infested with cockroaches have a much higher incidence of severe asthma than children whose living quarters are cockroach-free. In fact, much of the current explosion of asthma cases in the inner city can be directly traced to a hard-to-control cockroach population. Being born during the winter seems to increase the severity of a child's reaction to cockroach allergen, probably because of the increased hours spent indoors.

Parents who smoke, during pregnancy or any time after, put their children at a significantly greater risk of developing asthma as well.

DIAGNOSING ASTHMA

Asthma can be very mild, or it can be severe. Generally, doctors consider asthma to be mild if a child has two or fewer brief episodes per week. A child's asthma is considered to be moderate if there are more than two episodes a week. For children with severe asthma, life can hold occasional periods of easy breathing but is marked by frequent, severe flares.

Is It Asthma?

Some cases of asthma are plain as plain can be: the child coughs and wheezes upon vigorous exercise and exposure to cold air, experiences difficulty during high pollen and mold seasons, and has experienced more recurrent symptoms ever since the family installed wall-to-wall carpeting.

Other cases, of which there are many, require a bit more sleuthing on the clinician's part. The signs and symptoms of asthma are many and various. What's more, asthma can present like other diseases. In infants and very young children, what was once diagnosed as pneumonia or bronchiolitis (a disease of the lower respiratory tract with the cough and wheezing similar to those in asthma) is now recognized to be asthma.

Because asthma is becoming increasingly common in young children, and prompt, early treatment is so vital to a child's health, most doctors are now taking the approach that if it seems as if it could be asthma, asthma should be the prime suspect.

In general, doctors will make a diagnosis of asthma if the child has experienced difficulty in breathing—from coughing to wheezing to a general feeling of chest tightness—on several occasions; experiences some relief when treated with asthma medications; and is not suffering from any other illness (cystic fibrosis, let's say) that would produce the same symptoms.

Asthma can manifest itself as a cough, chest tightness, wheezing, breathlessness, or a combination of all four. But reaching a true asthma diagnosis can be tricky. Many babies who wheeze do not have asthma, and not every child with asthma wheezes! To reach a diagnosis of asthma, a doctor will probably ask you these questions:

• Does your child seem to be short of breath while doing everyday activities, or get winded much more easily than other children when playing? Some children, of course, have less stamina than others, and everyone huffs and puffs now and then. But if you notice what seems to be a substantial difference—your child riding a trike for ten minutes or so at a time, while friends happily ride all afternoon—it is worth mentioning.

• Do you ever hear your child wheeze, or hear a whistling sound when he or she is breathing? Noisy breathing from the chest can mean many things, but asthma is the most common.

• Does your child always seem to have excess phlegm that can't be explained by a cold? People with asthma produce more mucus than average.

• Does your child begin coughing after laughing hard, crying, raising his or her voice, or running around? If your child has a several-minutes-long coughing episode after every tickle-fest, or begins coughing within minutes of beginning to cry, that should raise a red flag.

• Does your child complain of discomfort in the chest, without evidence of an illness? Young children don't have the words for "chest tightness" or "chest congestion," but they often will complain that their chest hurts.

• Does your child wake often at night, usually at the same times? It could be separation anxiety. It also could be asthma. Asthma is worse at night.

• Does it seem to be hard for your child to take a deep breath? Although asthma makes *exhaling* difficult, you can't take a deep breath when your lungs are already fairly full.

• Does your child seem to have less get-up-and-go than most children? Does he or she seem to avoid exercise? Does your child seem to require a lot more rest than most children? As anyone who's suffered a bad head cold can attest to, not breathing well can really wear you out.

• Is your child not growing well or gaining enough weight? Children with untreated asthma tend not to seem as robust as others.

• Does your child begin coughing upon exposure to cold air, or while being outside during the spring and fall? Although asthma affects people year-round, spring's pollens and fall's molds are notorious triggers. If there does seem to be an environmental trigger, have you noticed a pattern?

• Does your child cough or wheeze after eating certain foods? Asthma is a common allergic reaction.

ASTHMA THROUGHOUT LIFE

If your child is going to develop asthma, you generally know it by the time he or she is seven years old. But that's only *generally*; asthma can show up at any time in life, from infancy through old age. The good news is that children who have had asthma since a very young age—age two and below—may get some real relief at around age five. A growth spurt in the bronchial tubes, providing a bit more "breathing room," plus a general tendency to not catch quite so many colds, can make life a lot easier. The teenage years are also important for children suffering from asthma. Some children seem to miraculously "outgrow" their asthma in puberty. (It may reappear later in life, but don't let that stop you from enjoying those wheeze-free years.) Unfortunately, if asthma is not outgrown in puberty, it probably will continue later in life. And while more boys than girls suffer with asthma as children—more than twice as many, in fact—more boys also tend to outgrow their asthma in puberty. By the end of the teenage years, the number of boys and girls with asthma is about the same. As adults, slightly more women than men have asthma.

Overall, children who have allergy-triggered asthma that began when they were under two years old, who continue to suffer from their allergies in adulthood, and who have frequent asthma episodes are the ones who will be dealing with asthma for the long haul. How hard a time they have of it, however, is very much within our control. Avoidance of the asthma triggers whenever possible, daily preventive treatment, prompt attention to symptoms, and a regular review of medication can keep virtually all children with asthma at the top of their game. In fact, many Olympic athletes have dealt with asthma for much of their lives. Keeping a child with asthma healthy is a blend of common sense, good medical guidance, careful observation, and experience. The key words are *avoidance*, *prevention*, and *treatment*. Remember, asthma is a disease of degrees: you *do* get some warning that a flare is about to begin. The goal in managing asthma is to prevent it when you can; catch it early and treat it promptly when you can't prevent the flare.

GUIDELINES FOR PREVENTING ASTHMA FLARES

The table on pages 301–2 lists some common causes of asthma flares and what you can do to try to prevent a full-blown episode from occurring. You'll be successful many times, but other times you won't. That's the nature of the beast. There's no way you'll be able to keep your child from catching a cold or two each winter or overdoing it on the playing field now and then. Here are some suggestions to keep your child as healthy as possible.

• Consider a yearly flu shot (provided your child is not allergic to eggs). Coming down with the flu can greatly exacerbate a child's asthma.

• Treat nasal symptoms promptly. The constant drip, drip, drip of that seemingly innocent case of the sniffles can trigger an asthma flare in your child. And remember that children with nasal allergies are much more likely to develop sinus infections than those who are not allergic.

• Try allergen immunotherapy (allergy shots) if your child is troubled by asthma for most of the year or cannot avoid certain asthma-provoking allergens.

• Cut down your child's incidence of colds by communicating the importance of washing hands with soap several times during the day, and keeping the hands away from the face.

• Protect your child from all forms of smoke, from cigarettes to wood-burning stoves and fireplaces. (Cigarette smoke is a hazard to *all* children.)

• Be vigilant about environmental allergens. Children with asthma most often react to dust mites, mold, pollen, cockroaches, and animal dander. See chapter 31, "Environmental Allergies," for techniques to bring indoor pollution levels way down.

• Remember that an older child or child in day care spends one-third of the day out of the home. When at all possible, become familiar with your child's school environment, both to identify possible asthma triggers (carpeting, strong odors, a freshly painted classroom, a new gym floor, pets in the classroom, lots of dust collectors, a musty smell) and to see simple ways the environment can be modified to protect your child's health.

IF YOUR CHILD'S ASTHMA FLARES:	YOU CAN PREVENT OR MINIMIZE IT BY:
Upon exposure to cold air	Wrapping a scarf around the nose and mouth in cold weather; breathing through the nose
During vigorous exercise	Starting the exercise slowly, encouraging activities such as swimming (the warm, moist air of an indoor pool is a boon for children with asthma) or moderate hiking, or, under your doctor's guidance, pre-treating your child with a bronchodilator directly before the activity
During an illness	Washing hands regularly, particularly upon returning home from public places; avoiding contact with sick playmates or family members; eating a well-balanced diet, drinking lots of fluids, and getting

	enough rest; getting a flu shot if your doctor recommends one
During the spring	Keeping all windows shut during the pollen season, using the air conditioner for cooling if necessary; keeping outdoor activity to a minimum on windy days and days with a high pollen count; taking a bath and washing hair every night, or even as soon as your child is inside for the evening
During the fall	Keeping all windows shut, using the air conditioner for cooling if necessary; avoiding fall yardwork such as raking leaves; absolutely avoiding areas where leaf blowers are being used

TREATING ASTHMA

Many of us believe that when it comes to treating an illness, the least amount of medication is the best amount of medication. And in most circumstances, that is indeed the case: a cold or the flu responds just as readily to lots of rest, warm liquids, and an aspirin-substitute as it does to loads of over-the-counter remedies; a garden-variety stomach bug can generally be as well controlled by a bland, starchy diet and plenty of fluids as it can by medicines. But asthma doesn't work that way. Regular and proper use of the medication prescribed by your health care professional is the best way to maintain your child's respiratory health and restore it when a flare-up occurs.

Asthma medications fall into two distinct categories: those that control inflammation with the goal of preventing an episode from occurring, and those that bring quick relief when an episode is under way.

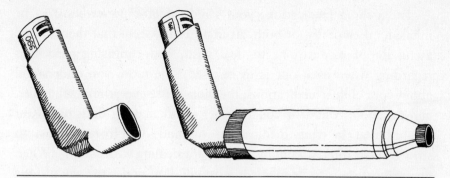

Quick-relief inhalers may be used on their own (left), which requires coordinating breath with delivery of medicine; or with a spacer (right), which is the preferred method for young children.

The most common medications for long-term use are:

- Cromolyn sodium (Intal)
- Inhaled corticosteroids such as Pulmocort Turbuhaler, Beclovent, Vanceril, AeroBid, Flovent, and Azmacort
- Oral corticosteroids such as Prelone, Pediapred, Medrol, Deltasone, and Prednisonel
- Leukotriene modifiers such as Singulair and Accolate
- Long-acting beta 2 agonists such as Serevant, Serevent Diskus, Volmax, and Preventil Repetabs (this last not for children under age six)
- Nedocromil sodium (Tilade)

The most common "rescue" medications (used during a flare-up) are:

- Short-acting inhaled beta 2 agonists, such as albuterol (Airet, Proventil, Ventolin), bitolterol (Tornalate), levalbuterol (Xopenex), and pirbuterol (Maxair)
- A short "burst" (three to ten days) of the oral corticosteroids featured above
- Ipratropium bromide (Atrovent)

The asthma medications your child's doctor prescribes may be inhaled, taken orally, or both. At first, it may seem that there are an awful lot of medications to deal with, and confusing guidelines regarding when each one is to be used. The more you understand about your child's medications, the more sense everything will make, and the more confident you will feel about making decisions. Rest assured that layering medications on and off—from mildest to strongest—is often a winning strategy for dealing with asthma. When the medication is to be inhaled, most children under the age of four use a nebulizer, a forced-air machine that turns liquid medicine into a mist. (Some children can use an inhaler with an aerochamber and mask—a method most often used for inhaled steroids—but the delivery of medication isn't as good.) Some children use their nebulizer with a mask that directs the mist into their nose and mouth. Others

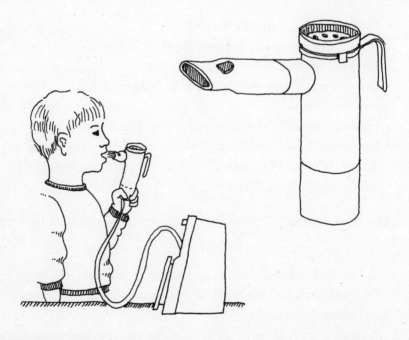

The nebulizer's aerochamber turns liquid medication into a fine mist for inhalation. The mist may be inhaled as shown. Very young children may do better using a face mask with their nebulizer.

prefer to do without the mask and have the nebulizer cup held at about mouth level so that the mist is easily inhaled as it rises. (This is perfectly effective, although some children complain about the mist getting into their eyes.) Depending on how much medicine you need to put in the cup, "nebulizing" your child can take from five to twenty minutes or so.

Your child's doctor will tell you what medication to use for which symptoms, how much to use, and when to use it. If you are confused, ask for as much clarification as you need. Handling asthma *can* be confusing, and everyone, doctors included, knows it. Don't be embarrassed to ask as many questions as you feel are necessary, even "silly" ones. But once you've asked all your questions and gotten your answers, *write down what your medical professional says and abide by it!*

The National Institutes of Health estimates that at least 100 million people worldwide suffer from asthma—and their numbers are rapidly increasing in developed nations. Over 4.8 million children in the United States alone are affected. But with proper controls (avoiding allergenic food and environments) and the right medicine given at the right time, most of those children can lead perfectly normal lives. Your child can too!

30

ATOPIC DERMATITIS (ECZEMA)

Dry, rashy, red skin that can weep, ooze, thicken, and crust. Itching beyond imagining. Days consumed with trying not to scratch and nights fractured by discomfort. "Oh," people will say kindly but dismissively, "but it's just eczema." To eczema sufferers, there's no "just" about it. Eczema, like the common cold, is one of those conditions that seldom arouses any reaction greater than mild sympathy from nonsufferers, but it can make you miserable down to your very core if you or your child are the one afflicted.

Eczema is thought to occur in 1 to 4 percent of all children in the United States. Although the exact cause is not known, there's no denying an allergic link in the majority of cases. Most children with eczema have inherited a tendency toward allergy from one or both parents. If you or your spouse has asthma, hay fever, food allergies, environmental allergies, or eczema, you've passed the atopic (allergenic) gene on to your child. Approximately 75 percent of all children with eczema go on to develop hay fever, asthma, or both.

If you pay careful attention, you may be able to eventually figure out what your child's eczema trigger is, whether it is a particular food or an environmental allergen such as dust, pollen, mold, or animal dander. (Or even all of the above.) Skin testing may also help you identify particular triggers. Some children are virtually symptom-free when the trigger is removed. If the trigger is a food (egg is a common culprit), the child may do extremely well following an elimination diet. For others, the eczema seems to be chronic. There will be times when it seems to be under control and times when it flares up, with little discernible rhyme or reason. This second type is debilitating and exhausting for all concerned, but there are some things you can do to make it less so. You'll find some tips in the "Treating Eczema" section of this chapter.

As with any itchy skin condition—chicken pox through mosquito bites—scratching does little good but can cause great harm. In many cases of eczema, it's the very act of scratching the itch that causes the distinctive rash. And once the rash has established itself, the skin is vulnerable to secondary infections. (Children with eczema are highly vulnerable to herpes infections, so be careful to avoid people with cold sores and chicken pox.) What's more, scratching can lead to more histamine release in the skin, which makes the itching even worse.

Unfortunately, babies and very small children can't be expected not to scratch something that itches, and you certainly don't want to set up a power struggle on that front. The best thing to do is keep

---

Keep Your Child Comfy

Children with eczema have such sensitive skin that virtually anything less than optimal conditions can trigger an itchy, rashy flare. In general, you can reduce the chances of this happening by avoiding:

- Wool, nylon, and clothing that binds or does not "breathe"
- Hot water, which actually has a dehydrating effect on the skin
- Soap, detergents, and solvents
- Overheating, sweating, and high humidity
- Dust, dirt, and newsprint

your child's nails (and your own) as short as possible, and dress your child in soft, comfortable clothing that completely covers the afflicted areas. Some physicians feel that using a soap product such as Ivory Snow instead of a detergent is easier on children's skin. At night, it's a good idea to put your child in footed pajamas with mittens (or even cotton socks) sewn onto the sleeves so they cannot be removed. (If your child needs to suck his or her thumb to fall asleep, you can simply cut an opening in the thumb area.)

It's important to know that kids with eczema do not regulate body temperature normally. They always seem to be hot or, conversely, always complain of being cold. They may sweat a lot or hardly at all. Not infrequently, their perception of how hot or cold it feels can be far off the mark from what others in the family feel. This can lead to a battle of wills, with a parent insisting that the child can't possibly be hot (or cold) at this particular temperature. But within reason, here's one time when the path of least resistance is the wisest one to take. Try to avoid extreme temperature changes, and then let your child's comfort be your guide. Although you may feel you need a turtleneck and sweater indoors on a chilly winter day, your child may feel miserably overheated in anything more than a T-shirt. And if he or she insists on sweatpants and a sweatshirt when the rest of the world is running around in shorts, try not to make too big a deal of it. The more comfortable your child is, the happier you all will be.

Children who suffer from severe outbreaks of eczema, with a substantial amount of broken skin, can be exceptionally thirsty during these episodes. That's because the skin plays a vital role in holding body fluid. When a great deal of the skin's surface is open, extra fluid is lost through evaporation. This isn't dangerous in and of itself, assuming that the child drinks enough to avoid becoming dehydrated. But when an outbreak is this severe, it's important to treat it promptly. All too quickly and too often, what starts out as garden-variety eczema can turn into a nasty bacterial infection (*Staphylococcus aureus* colonization of skin is all too common in children with eczema) or a breeding ground for viral infections such as warts and herpes. If you see any signs that a bacterial infection is starting, consult your health care professional at once.

TREATING ECZEMA

Eczema cannot be "cured," but it can usually be fairly well managed. And in nine out of ten cases, Nature lends a helping hand: 50 percent of all children with eczema completely outgrow their condition by the end of early childhood, and 40 percent will be left with only minor or occasional problems. The remaining 10 percent will continue to fight the good fight throughout adulthood.

In the meantime, there are some simple, straightforward measures to take that can go a long way toward alleviating discomfort and keeping infection at a minimum. To alleviate discomfort, the most important thing of all is to establish and stick to a daily skin care routine of soaks and creams. Some children will get relief from just one bath a day. Others need three or more—ask your health care professional. If you feel soap is absolutely necessary, it's best to stick with mild brands such as Dove, Basis, or Neutrogena. Sally Noone, R.N., of the Jaffe Institute for Food Allergy at Mount Sinai School of Medicine, offers the following bath-time tips:

- Bathwater should be pleasantly warm only. Water that is too hot can increase itching. Plus, if your child has open areas in the skin, bathwater may burn. Try adding a half cup of table salt or Dome-Boro powder (the commercial name for Burow's solution) to the bathwater.

- Water should be deep enough to reach the child's stomach when sitting. Close supervision is essential whenever a young child is in the tub. Keep the neck and shoulders covered with a wet towel (as a shawl) during the soak, rewetting as needed.

- Holes cut into an old washcloth to make a mask can be helpful in keeping the face soaked as well.

- Provide bath toys to make it fun. Your child needs to soak *at least thirty minutes* to obtain the proper hydration of the skin.

- Reading books together or listening to tapes (be sure to keep all electrical equipment far from the tub and out of your child's reach!) during the bath can make this a special time for you and your child.

• Once out of the tub, barely pat the child dry before applying a moisturizer. Vaseline, Vanicream, Unibase, Acid Mantle, Complex 15, and Aquaphor are frequently used. Do not use lotion, as these are water-based. Your child's skin may seem softer with a particular product, or one may feel more comfortable. Any of these will help seal in the moisture from the soaking bath.

• Mild steroid creams or ointments (such as triamcinolone or flu-ocinolone) may have been prescribed for your child. They should be applied to areas of the body with redness or rash. Only 1 percent hydrocortisone should be used on the face.

If a young child needs relief but you cannot supervise a bath (or your child is getting cranky and wants nothing more than to watch a video), a "spa" treatment of warm soaks in wet cloths can also be very effective, both for controlling the itching and relaxing your child. Lay a rubber sheet or plastic on the surface your child will be lying on, and wrap your child up in towels soaked with either plain warm water or DomeBoro powder mixed with water as directed on the label. Cover your child with a washable blanket or quilt to keep warm. Leave the towels on for at least thirty minutes, then immediately apply the creams. This may be done three to four times a day for up to five days, or until the eczema flare subsides.

Some children with eczema also have seborrheic dermatitis—heavy scalp flaking that itches, scales, and looks generally unsightly. This happens when skin cells on the scalp reproduce themselves too quickly and are then flaked off. There are shampoos on the market such as Sebulex (salicylic soap) that can be of great help, but consult your health care professional before using them on your child. If you are given the green light to use a shampoo of this kind, you should wash your child's hair daily, leaving the lather on the scalp for at least five minutes. Once the flaking seems to be improving, you need only use the special shampoo twice a week.

MEDICATIONS FREQUENTLY USED FOR ECZEMA

Although no drug can cure eczema, there are different types that can help you manage the symptoms and secondary problems that may occur. Unfortunately, no vitamin supplements, shots, or oils have been proven to give any sort of relief—and allergy shots may indeed only make the situation worse. Depending on your child's needs, your physician may prescribe none, one, or all of these recognized effective medications at any given time.

• *Antihistamines.* As you know from dealing with food allergies, antihistamines block the negative effects of histamine production: nasal congestion or runniness, itchy eyes, swelling, and in the case of eczema, itchy skin. Unfortunately, antihistamines are only truly useful if they are already in your child's bloodstream when the allergic reaction occurs. If your child's physician thinks that antihistamines are the way to go, he or she will probably put your child on a regular dosing schedule, to keep the medication at a constant level in your child's body. Some children will experience sleepiness as a result of taking antihistamines. A few may go the opposite way and become hyper. Give your doctor's office a call to report any troublesome side effects.

• *Antipruretics.* These "anti-itching" medications are used to prevent scratching during sleep.

• *Antibiotics.* Children with eczema often have infection on their skin. And the more infection they have, the more inflamed and itchy their skin becomes. Antibiotics treat the infection and by doing so help contain the rash and discomfort. There are several antibiotics your health care professional may prescribe if this is the case with your child. Be sure to give the proper dosages for the specified amount of time to get the medicine's full effectiveness.

• *Corticosteroids.* Nothing works quite so well as these drugs when you need them, but as they are the medical equivalent of calling out the cavalry, they are generally prescribed sparingly and for brief periods. Corticosteroids are cortisone medications that can be taken as pills or syrup. They block inflammation and allergic responses for as long as your child is taking them. You may notice some side effects such as increased activity level and increased appetite while your child is on this medication. (If your child is of school age, it would not be a bad idea to alert the teacher.) Some children have the pleasant side effect of a heightened good mood. These are powerful drugs with potentially serious side effects, so use them with care and only as prescribed by your child's doctor.

31

ENVIRONMENTAL ALLERGIES

Environmental allergies are those caused by outside agents: the pollen in the air, the flying dander from the cat, the mold spores on autumn leaves, the dust on the bookcase, even the strong odors given off by new carpeting, the rubberized floor at the gym, or perfume.

The bad news about environmental allergens is that they can be present in mass quantities without any visible detection. The same home that so pleasantly shelters your beloved family and cherished possessions can also be home to a denizen of unsavory microscopic life-forms that can make just taking a deep breath pure misery. There's a certain amount of innocence we all lose when we learn what's truly living in our pillows and on our bathroom tile. (Once I gazed upon a dust mite, I was never able to look at velvet-draped Victorian-style rooms in quite the same way, and you probably won't be able to, either.) But like so much in life, a small loss in innocence can bring a proportionate measure of wisdom. And in this case, with that wisdom may also come a substantial improvement in your child's health.

DUST ALLERGY

It may manifest itself as a constant runny or stuffy nose, eczema, or asthma. But whatever the symptoms, house dust—even if you are a gold-star housekeeper—is a very common cause of children's environmental allergies. If your allergist suspects that your child has a problem with dust, he or she will be able to tell for certain with a simple skin test or blood test.

The house dust that settles on your shelves and blinds and into your curtains and rugs is an unappealing mix of many substances, many of which may cause an allergic reaction in a susceptible child. But for the most part, when children are allergic to dust, what they are reacting to are the waste products produced by a microscopic creature called a dust mite. Seen under an electron microscope, the dust mite looks like a hairy little tick, although its closest relative is actually the spider. Each of these strange tiny creatures produces about twenty waste particles a day, and each female can produce up to fifty baby dust mites about every three weeks. So it's easy to see how a small dust problem can become a big one in just a matter of months—especially because even after a dust mite dies, its allergy-producing waste products remain.

There's no pretty way of putting this: dust mites live on a diet of human skin flakes. They need us—and to a limited extent, we need them too. But don't worry; even when we've done everything in our power to rid ourselves of dust, we will still have plenty of dust mites to go around. Dust mites love a soft, warm, humid environment, particularly in bedding, carpet, stuffed toys, quilts, curtains, and upholstered furniture. And once they've settled in, they're there to stay. So the key to taming a dust problem is to either remove the dust mites' place of residence or make it not so appealing anymore.

Dust-proofing Your Home

When your child is allergic to the waste products produced by dust mites, it's time to start loving a clean, fresh look. Strictly speaking,

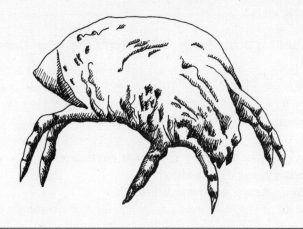

These strange microscopic creatures called dust mites live on a diet of skin flakes and are related to spiders. Their waste products are the culprit in allergy symptoms.

knickknacks, stacks of books, dried flowers, throw pillows, heavy upholstery, wall-to-wall carpeting, wool area rugs, and sumptuously draped fabrics are the enemy. Bare floors, open windows (assuming that pollen from grass, flowers, or trees isn't a problem), washable throw rugs, and a light hand with decorative objects are your friends. But unlike food allergies, where complete and total avoidance is the only route to health, environmental allergies give you the option of a middle ground. You know you've found it when your child's symptoms either go away or significantly abate.

Although it would be ideal if every one of us with a dust-allergic child could merrily pull up the carpeting, bid adieu to the window treatments, and replace all of our cushy sofas with plain wood or leather and chrome, few of us are in a position or mind-set to take such drastic measures throughout our homes. While major offenders like wall-to-wall carpeting and heavy drapes should go if at all possible (or should be regularly treated with a miticide if not), the room that's most important—and is easiest to control—is your child's bedroom.

Research has shown that minimizing your child's exposure to dust in his or her bedroom is the key link in tackling a dust allergy.

Controlling Dust Allergy: What Works and What Doesn't

Keeping the household humidity as close to 50 percent as possible during the winter and using air conditioners in the summer are simple measures that are highly effective to combat the misery of a dust-related allergy. Other important measures are:

- Staying with bare floors or stripping as much carpeting as possible, especially in your child's bedroom
- Replacing curtains and drapes with blinds
- Encasing pillows, mattresses, box springs, and quilts in allergen-proof covers

Less effective or not proven to be effective are:

- Chemically treating carpets with benzyl benzoate
- Tannic acid
- Air cleaners

Sometimes recommended for spraying onto carpets and upholstery, tannic acid can render the dust mite waste products less allergenic, but it generally does not have a long-lasting effect. As for air cleaners, while they are very effective for animal dander (which is so small and light it remains airborne for hours), they are not particularly necessary to combat dust. Dust mite allergens are larger and heavier, so they generally settle in under an hour.

Because not only does your child spend over a third of the day there, bedrooms are a dust mite's favorite abode. Box springs, mattresses, pillows, and quilts are all wonderfully conducive to dust mite health and reproduction. Add carpeting, stuffed animals, curtains, books, and wall hangings, and you've got a virtual dust mite nirvana. (And you thought you were creating that delightful environment for your *child*, didn't you.) Help is at hand. The worksheet and diagram that appear at the end of this section, used with the kind permission of Allergy Control Products in Ridgefield, Connecticut (phone: [800] 422-DUST), cover all the bases. Talk to your child's allergist about how many of these measures are appropriate for your child. Everyone agrees that mattresses and box spring covers, pillow covers, and hot water washes for bedding are a must. Removing or regularly treating carpeting and curtains is also a must. Simple measures such as keeping closet doors closed and keeping books and toys in closed cabinets can make a surprisingly big difference. Other helpful strategies are as follows:

- Wash your child's stuffed animals in hot water every two weeks, or, if you can't bear the thought of that, kill those pesky dust mites by placing the stuffed animals in a plastic bag and putting them in the freezer during the day.
- Dust all surfaces at least twice a week with a pretreated cloth, damp rag, or damp mop to really "catch" the dust, not just move it from place to place.
- Keep your child out of rooms that are being dusted and vacuumed while they're being cleaned and for at least twenty minutes after. You'd be amazed at how much dust gets in the air even when the best cleaning methods are used.
- Wash all of your child's sheets, pillowcases, and blankets or blanket covers in water that's at least 130 degrees. Dust mites are impervious to soap and water, and dryers don't get hot enough to kill them. If you have lowered your water temperature, you can add a teapot of boiling water to the load of laundry or have your child's bedding washed at a launderette (be sure to use hot wash).

All this being said, the bedroom of a dust-allergic child can look every bit as warm and friendly as any other child's room. And as a side benefit, because children who can't tolerate dust must of necessity cut down on clutter, their bedrooms can and should be soothingly neat and well ordered. These simple decorating tricks can easily and inexpensively turn even the most sparsely furnished bedroom into a happy place for a child to live.

- Color is king! Choose a theme for your child's room—astronauts, dinosaurs, ballet dancers, the rain forest—and follow it through with a wallpaper border and coordinating paint. If you're artistic (or are lucky to be in the good graces of an artistic friend), you might even want to paint a mural or two on the walls. While lots of framed pictures are a no-no unless you are truly committed to high-level dusting, beautiful paint and/or wallpaper doesn't attract any more dust than a plain white wall would.

• Paint isn't just for walls. If the bare floors in your child's room are less than lovely, consider sanding them smooth, then covering them with a few coats of floor paint. Some people use just one solid color, others get creative with stencils, and still others paint on rug patterns, a bed of flowers, a race track, or whatever their imaginations decide. If you have lovely hardwood floors, show them off with a new coat of varnish, then add a few small washable rugs for warmth.

• Unfinished furniture can also be painted to continue the theme of the room or just to color-coordinate. Not only is it inexpensive, you can simply apply a fresh coat in a new color when your child's taste changes.

• Even a dust-free bed can be a deliciously warm and cozy bed. Loads of pillows are fine so long as they are first encased in allergen-impermeable covers. A nice fluffy quilt encased in a similar cover is also fine, provided you wash the duvet cover in hot water every two weeks. And I've been most pleasantly surprised at how well major manufacturers' sheets have held up to the hot water treatment year after year. Go for those colors—they'll take a beating before they fade.

• If curtain-less windows seem too bare, you can create a warmer look with a small ruffle or rectangular cornice made of fabric you can wash in hot water each week.

• Although books and toys—dust catchers all—should be kept to a minimum, a glass-front cabinet that is kept closed can be used to store and display some precious possessions. For more rough-and-tumble kids, a storage system made of closed plastic containers can also be used. The idea here is to have as little dust in the air as possible when your child is sleeping.

DUST ALLERGEN AVOIDANCE WORKSHEET
(in accordance with National Asthma Education Program
National Heart, Lung and Blood Institute • National Institutes of Health)

PRIMARY OBJECTIVES

_____ 1. Encase pillows in allergen-impermeable covers or wash every two weeks in hot water.

_____ 2. Encase mattress (and box spring) in allergen-impermeable covers.

_____ 3. Wash blankets every two weeks in hot water.

_____ 4. Encase comforters in allergen-impermeable covers or wash every two weeks in hot water.

_____ 5. Wash bed linen (sheets and pillowcases) in hot water every two weeks.

_____ 6. Remove bedroom carpeting if at all possible.

Notes:_____

_____

_____

SECONDARY OBJECTIVES

_____ 1. If unable to remove carpeting:
    a. denature allergen using tannic acid
    b. use a miticide to kill mites

_____ 2. Maintenance of carpet:
    a. vacuum weekly wearing a mask
    b. clean carpet with dry powdered cleaner to help remove allergen
    c. upgrade vacuum cleaner filtration (filters, bags, HEPA vacuum cleaner)

_____ 3. If hot air heating system:
    a. close vents and use electric heater in bedroom
    b. use electrostatic filter on vent opening
    c. use central electrostatic filter system

_____ 4. Remove dust collectors.

Notes:_____

_____

THINGS TO CONSIDER

_____ 1. Systems to reduce humidity:
    a. air-conditioning
    b. dehumidification units

_____ 2. HEPA room air cleaners

Notes:_____

_____

_____

Physician's Signature   Date

DUST CONTROL IN THE BEDROOM

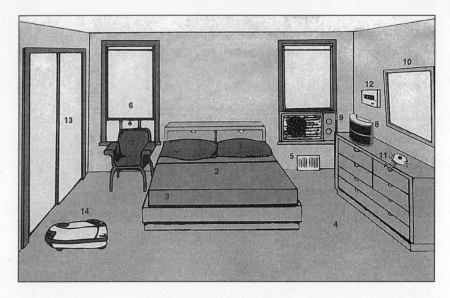

1. Encase the pillows in zippered, allergen-impermeable covers, or wash pillows in hot water every two weeks. Covers such as Allergy Control Covers which permit perspiration vapor transmission will be most comfortable.

2. Encase the mattress and box spring in zippered, allergen-impermeable encasings. If there is more than one bed in the room, all should be encased. Covers such as Allergy Control Covers which permit perspiration vapor transmission will be most comfortable.

3. Wash all bedding—blankets, sheets, pillowcases, and mattress pad if used—in hot water (130°) every two weeks. Avoid wool and down blankets. Comforters can be encased in allergen-impermeable interliners with decorative cover or washed every two weeks.

4. Remove all carpeting. If this is not possible, apply a solution to inactivate allergen and/or a miticide to kill dust mites.

5. Cover hot air vents with filters to clean the air at point-of-entry, or close the vents and use an electric radiator.

6. Avoid heavy curtains and blinds. Use window shades instead. If curtains are used, launder them frequently.

7. Use wipeable furniture (wood, plastic, vinyl, or leather) in place of upholstered furniture.

8. HEPA air cleaners can remove airborne allergen particles. Be sure to choose the appropriate model for your room size. Air cleaners should not be placed where their exhaust can disturb settled dust from carpets and nearby furnishings.

9. Use air conditioners to prevent the high heat and humidity which stimulate mite growth. Special filters can be added to help trap the airborne allergens. Use a dehumidifier to help reduce humidity levels.

10. Avoid dust collectors, such as wall pennants, macrame hangings, and throw pillows. Remove or machine wash stuffed toys.

11. Wear a well-fitting face mask when doing housecleaning and other chores. Clean drawers, closets, and surfaces with a treated cloth.

12. Avoid over-humidification if using a humidifier in the winter. Mites grow best at 75–80 percent relative humidity and cannot live under 50 percent humidity. The ideal relative humidity is 40–50 percent. Use a humidity gauge to monitor levels.

13. Keep all clothing in a closet, with the door shut.

14. Use a vacuum cleaner with high allergen containment. A multilayer dust bag and exhaust filter will reduce escape of allergen.

MOLDS

Many food-allergic children will develop a runny nose, eczema, or wheezing when they're not eating anything at all. They're just happily playing in the lovely new playroom you've recently added—fully *carpeted*, freshly painted, *in the basement*. Or they're running around *outside* on a beautiful *fall* day, jumping into the occasional pile of *leaves*. Or they've spent a rainy day being mother's helper: cleaning out *closets*, sorting *laundry*, cleaning the *kitchen* and *bathrooms*. Any one of these activities is likely to trigger a reaction in a child who is allergic to mold.

If your first response is "not in *my* house!" think again. Unless you live in a zero-humidity home in an area where there's always a blanket of snow on the ground, there's no avoiding mold and mildew. With over 10,000 varieties and a billions-year-old capacity to adapt to virtually any circumstances they find themselves in, these microscopic fungi and their spores are among the most populous organisms on Earth—more prevalent by far than pollen, and far less affected by seasonal changes. There are almost always mold spores in the air, which are more than happy to waft into your house and begin colonizing at the first hospitable area, joining millions of relatives who've already set up camp.

Taken from a human perspective, this has its good and bad points. Molds live on plant or animal matter, which they eat by decomposing. So while you may not welcome the mold on your bread, you or someone near and dear has no doubt been the beneficiary of antibiotics, which are made from mold. And while the mildew on your bathroom ceiling is cause for consternation, mildew's cousin the mushroom not only is a tasty addition to your omelette, but also helps clear the forests of decaying wood. Some molds are highly toxic; others are vital to growing healthy crops. But the simple fact remains that molds are here to stay. If our children are allergic to them, all we can do is control their growth and our children's exposure to them.

As anyone who has ever dealt with damp towels in the summertime knows, mold and mildew thrive in a warm, humid environment. Bathrooms and basements are their favorite abodes, but they're happy to take up residence under your refrigerator, on your leftovers, in your hampers and your closets, on your walls, in your garbage cans, and on just about every other surface in your home. And as with dust mites, just because you don't see them doesn't mean they aren't there. Helping a mold-allergic child means not only paying particular attention to the areas mold prefers but looking at your home environment as a whole.

If you live in the suburbs or the country, you need to be particularly careful about mold outside: compost piles and grass clippings in spring and summer; raked leaves and wooded areas in fall. In fact, most children with mold allergies will have their worst symptoms during the fall months, when the combination of often rainy conditions, generally mild weather, and decaying leaves and plant matter makes being a mold spore a truly fine thing. A freezing winter offers some relief. If you live in a climate where the weather is fairly warm and humid all year long, you have your work cut out for you—but you've no doubt been battling mildew for so long that you are sworn enemies already.

Indoors, the key is keeping the environment as dry as you can without undue discomfort. Most allergists agree that families with mold-allergic children should aim to keep the indoor environment at a maximum of 50 percent humidity. But, unless you live in an arid region, that's easier said than done. Your best bet is to go out and buy a few humidity gauges—they're quite inexpensive—and place them in strategic parts of your home. Don't be surprised to find readings of 70 percent humidity even during the winter months. Unfortunately, that's a comfortable environment not only for us humans but for the dust mites and mold spores we share our homes with as well. Simple measures to keep the humidity down include running the exhaust fan when you shower, running air conditioners and/or dehumidifiers in the summer, and not humidifying your home in the winter. This can be a delicate balancing act, as anyone knows who has welcomed the relief from coughs and croup a humidifier provides. Unless your child has a severe mold allergy, most health care professionals will endorse the limited use of a humidifier to get through a particularly bad bout of bronchitis or croup—nighttime use only, and only for a few days. But it's always best to check first.

Other major contributors to a mold problem in the home are carpets (particularly bathroom carpet and carpeted basements), foam rubber pillows and mattresses, and benign neglect in the refrigerator and laundry areas. (In other words, clean out the refrigerator regularly and put that damp laundry in the dryer ASAP.) See the following chart for specific guidelines on controlling mold, used by permission of Allergy Control Products.

MOLD CONTROL IN THE HOME

THROUGHOUT THE HOUSE

- Keep humidity low, 35 percent if possible, but in no case over 50 percent. Use a gauge to monitor relative humidity.
- Use an air conditioner or dehumidifier in times of high humidity, with the windows closed. Dehumidifiers must be emptied of water regularly, or connected to a constant drain. Air conditioners should be sprayed at the air intake with a mold killing spray if they develop a musty odor. Special air conditioner filters can be added to help trap the airborne allergens, and room air cleaners can help clear the air of mold spores.
- Very tightly insulated houses prevent the escape of moisture and thus encourage mold growth. Allow adequate ventilation.
- If using a humidifier in the winter, avoid over-humidification. If mold is present, rinse the interior of the unit with a dilute bleach solution. Some humidifiers prevent mold growth by a special heating process. Central humidifiers should be checked and cleaned frequently.
- Clean walls and ceilings and add mold inhibitor to paint before applying.
- Window condensation can lead to moisture and mold growth on the window frame.
- Although indoor plants are not a major source of indoor mold spores, it is prudent to limit the number of houseplants.
- Mold is present on the bark of wood. If using a fireplace or woodburning stove, do not store firewood inside. Avoid live Christmas trees.

IN THE BEDROOM

- Follow steps to decrease dust exposure. Ideally, carpeting should be removed and mattresses encased in allergen-impermeable zippered covers.
- Avoid foam rubber pillows and mattresses, since they are particularly likely to become moldy.
- A dehumidifier or air conditioner can help reduce humidity.

- Mold grows in closets, which are damp and dark. Dry shoes and boots thoroughly before storing. Use a chemical moisture remover in closets and storage spaces to help prevent mold growth.
- Good-quality HEPA air cleaners can remove mold spores from the air.
- Convection heat units can make mold spores nonviable and help reduce the spread of mildew.

IN THE BATHROOM
- Use an exhaust fan or open window to remove humidity after showering. Use a squeegee to remove excess water from shower stall, tub, and tiles.
- Wash shower curtain, bathroom tiles, shower stall, tub, toilet tank, and tiles with mold-killing and mold-preventing solutions.
- Do not carpet the bathroom.

IN THE KITCHEN
- Use an exhaust fan to remove water vapor when cooking.
- Mold can grow in refrigerators, particularly around door gaskets. Empty water pans below self-defrosting refrigerators frequently. Remove spoiling foods immediately.
- Molds grow in garbage containers, which should be emptied frequently and kept clean.

IN THE LAUNDRY ROOM
- Vent the clothes dryer to the outdoors. Dry clothing immediately after washing.

IN THE BASEMENT
- Carpet and pad should not be laid on a concrete floor. Vinyl flooring is a better choice.
- Correct seepage or flooding problems, and remove any previously flooded carpet. If a dirt floor is present, cover with a plastic vapor barrier.
- Keep the basement free of dust, and remove moldy stored items.
- Add a paint mold inhibitor to paint, especially on brick or cinder-block walls.
- Allergic individuals should not have their bedroom on the basement level.

OUT OF DOORS
- Avoid cutting grass and raking leaves, or use a well-fitting face mask if these chores must be done by the allergic individual. Avoid exposure to soil, compost piles, sandboxes, hay, fertilizers, and barns. Prune or cut trees to avoid shading of the home. Eliminate vines.
- Correct drainage problems near the house, as pooled water greatly increases mold formation.
- Avoid camping or walking in the woods, where mold growth on rotted logs and other vegetation is high. Some mold spores are spread on dry and windy days, others at times of rainfall.

WORK AND MISCELLANEOUS ENVIRONMENTS
- Greenhouses, antiques shops, sleeping bags, summer cottages, and hotel rooms are sources of increased mold exposure. Automobile air conditioners may harbor mold.
- Occupational exposure to mold occurs in farmers, gardeners, bakers, brewers, florists, carpenters, mill workers, upholsterers, and paperhangers. Your allergist can offer specific recommendations.

ANIMAL ALLERGY

An allergic child can be allergic to any warm-blooded animal at all. In fact some frustrated animal lovers, allergic to the dander (skin flakes) produced by fur-bearing animals, have turned to keeping hedgehogs, only to find that many of them are allergic to the animal's saliva. (Apparently hedgehogs lick themselves a lot.) But when it comes to causing problems, cats are at the top of the pantheon. Cat allergen is found in both the dander and saliva of cats. Not only is this allergen particularly strong, it is extraordinarily small (one-tenth the size of a dust mite) and fiendishly difficult to get out of the environment. What's more, because cat allergen is extremely sticky and is carried on clothing, it can be found virtually anywhere you find people who own cats, including office buildings, public transportation, movie theaters, schools, stores, and all public places that cat owners visit. Cat dander is notoriously sticky; all it takes is one affectionate rub for a cat to deposit allergen on your clothing that you will take with you wherever you go that day. Fortunately, unless your child is exquisitely sensitive to cat allergen, chances are that none of these random (and basically unavoidable) exposures are likely to cause a reaction.

Allergies to small animals such as guinea pigs, rabbits, hamsters, and gerbils can usually be quelled by removing the animal from the home and effecting a thorough vacuuming and cleaning of the area in which they lived. Allergies to dogs can be handled in much the same way, though on a larger scale. But once you've got significant levels of cat allergen in your house, you're in it for the long haul.

The first and most important step is to remove the cat. If, for whatever reason, you cannot remove the cat from the household, you absolutely must remove the cat from your child's bedroom. Plus, your child's bedroom door must be kept closed at all times, including at night when your child is sleeping, to make sure the cat doesn't pay a silent surprise visit.

If there are air ducts leading to your child's room, they must be covered with a filter; cat allergens are highly mobile.

If You Can't Give Up Your Cat . . .

The best remedy for the symptoms of cat allergy is to find your pet a loving new home, then do a complete cleanup of your own home environment. (See text.) If that is unacceptable or not possible right now, you can try these measures. They should reduce but will not eliminate the problem.

• Confine your pet to the part of your home that is least likely to be frequented by your child: a den, home office, or dining room, for example. Bare floors are best, as they can be wiped down to remove allergens.

• If the cat is in a carpeted area, it's best to vacuum with a vacuum cleaner especially designed to contain allergens. If you choose not to buy one, at least use allergen-containment vacuum cleaner bags in your regular vacuum.

• Always wash your hands with warm soapy water after petting the cat, and try to avoid sitting on furniture or rugs that the cat sits on.

• Keep your windows open in the spring and summer (unless seasonal allergies are a problem) to let the dander out. When colder weather hits or when windows need to be closed, use a HEPA or ULPA air cleaner to trap these fiendishly tiny airborne allergens.

Like most microscopic environmental allergens, cat allergen presents the biggest problem when it becomes airborne, which it does at the rustle of a comforter, the tread of a foot on carpet, the shifting pressure of a sleeping body on a mattress. In other words, it doesn't take much. And even once a cat has been removed from the environment, it can take almost half a year for carpets to be relatively "clean" of cat allergen (unless you use special allergen-containment bags, vacuuming generally only scatters the allergen through the air) and many years for mattresses to be considered safe. Clearly, this is far too long for a child to suffer. The best course of action is to immediately pull up the carpeting in your child's room and encase his or her mattress in an allergen-impermeable cover. If, for any reason, you cannot remove the carpeting in the room, you can use one of the commercially available denaturing sprays to neutralize the allergen. (This would be a good move for every carpeted room in your home.) Every surface is suspect: scrub down the walls, use specially treated dust cloths for furniture, and thoroughly wash soft furnishings such as blankets, quilts, throw pillows, and throw rugs.

If your child is very allergic to cats, you may find that he or she has a reaction if a cat-owning friend or relative visits. There's enough cat allergen on the person's clothing alone to trigger a response. A friend of mine had this problem with a beloved baby-sitter. At first she thought it was the girl's perfume that was making her children wheeze, so the baby-sitter obligingly came unscented. When they finally figured out the cat connection, the baby-sitter showered and changed into a fresh outfit immediately before her expected arrival time.

In general, female cats and neutered males produce less allergen, but they still produce enough to make a child very sick. There is some evidence to suggest that washing the cat weekly to cut down on the amount of dander, urine, and dried saliva on the animal's skin may be effective, but it is not yet confirmed. If your child is suffering, it's certainly worth a try.

COCKROACHES

Yes, they are disgusting—and not just to look at, either. Did you know that a cockroach can live for up to ten days without its head? Its brain is divided among its body parts, so the only reason it dies is that without a head it can't drink. Aside from the obvious concerns of sanitation, cockroaches (more specifically, their body parts and waste products) are a leading cause of asthma and other allergic miseries in young children. Like all vermin, cockroaches are attracted to water and food: the water that collects in your sink from a drippy faucet, the crumbs on your kitchen table, an overflowing garbage can, or stray cookies in the cupboard. But as most every city dweller will tell you, cockroaches can turn up in even the cleanest households, fortified from a visit at your next-door neighbor's abode or brought along for the ride in your grocery bags. Even if you've never seen a cockroach in your present dwelling, if you live in an urban area you've got to assume they're out there and act accordingly.

Given their choice, cockroaches prefer a warm, humid climate, so once again the allergy-smart recommendation is to keep your home as close as possible to 50 percent humidity. Repair all pipes and faucets as soon as they start leaking. Breadstuffs and cereals that are kept in your cupboards should be in sealed plastic containers. An open package of food is an open invitation to a cockroach (who most likely has a large family or one on the way). Immediately wash all dishes after use, and rinse dishes well before putting them in the dishwasher. Keep your oven clean; in the winter especially, cockroaches are attracted to its warmth and grease spills. Empty your garbage can, and clean the area in which it is stored, on a regular basis.

With young children in the house, many of us feel wary about the poisons used by commercial exterminators. (Boric acid is safe and effective for use around older children, but you wouldn't want to run the risk of a toddler getting into it.) There are some preparations available, however, that are safe to use. Some people believe that bay leaves or cucumber rinds repel roaches, and they are certainly worth a try, particularly if your roach problem is modest. But if you are in the midst of a wide-scale invasion, you'll probably need something more lethal. Check in your local yellow pages, and you'll no doubt find a company that uses an organic compound. If you cannot find one, contact the local branch of the Environmental Protection Agency for ideas. The method you ultimately choose doesn't matter as much as the fact that you're tackling the problem. Cockroaches and allergic children are a bad combination, and the sooner you wipe out your vermin population, the better.

POLLEN

Pollen is how trees, grasses, and weeds reproduce; it is a microscopic reproductive cell these plants release into the air. In that sense, pollen

---

Treating Environmental Allergies

While prevention is always the preferred method of avoiding allergic symptoms, prevention isn't always feasible. There is no way to avoid exposure to outdoor allergens such as ragweed and pollen, for example, short of keeping your child under house arrest. Depending on your child's symptoms, your allergist may prescribe one or more of the following medications.

- For itchy eyes and nasal symptoms: antihistamines such as Benadryl, Claritin, or Zyrtec, and/or nasal sprays such as Nasonex or Rhinocort
- For asthma symptoms: an antihistamine (if nasal symptoms are present) to control mucus production, which can exacerbate asthma; *plus* expanded treatment with your child's regularly prescribed medication, perhaps used in conjunction with an inhaled steroid such as Pulmicort
- For skin symptoms: an antihistamine, plus topical creams if necessary. (See chapter 30 for helpful tips on soothing itchy skin.)

---

is an enormously good and necessary thing. But you don't need to ask children with pollen allergy how they feel when pollen season is at its height. The answer is plain: "yucky!" And because pollen is carried on the breeze, bright, sunny, windy days—perfect for kite flying, bike riding, and all-around cavorting—are generally more difficult for allergic children than rainy days, which wet the pollen down so it's not flying around in the air.

Depending on where you live in the United States, pollen can be a year-round misery or a seasonal one. In the Northeast there's very little pollen in the air in the wintertime, giving allergy sufferers a short break from that particular trigger. (Of course indoor allergens such as dust mites and mold abound, and viruses bearing colds and flu bring their own brand of misery.) But come springtime, with the arrival of those first tender green leaves, the air fills with tree pollen. Grass pollen hits in midsummer, and weed pollen is generally worst in the fall. Molds abound as well in the warm, humid air, making seasonal allergic rhinitis sufferers stuffy, sneezy, itchy, and even wheezy.

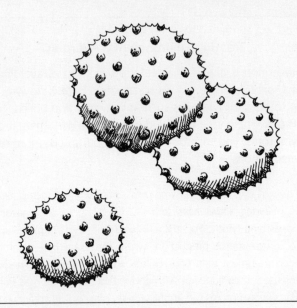

Without pollen we would have no grass, trees, flowers, or shrubs—but far fewer sneezes, rashes, and wheezes!

In warm climates and in the West, the pollen seasons usually start a good two to three months sooner, as early as February in many places. But a mild winter in the Northeast can cause the pollen season to start as early as March.

Many children are allergic to some pollens—ragweed and grass, let's say—but not others. Some kids are allergic to all pollens. Symptoms can be confined to itchy eyes or nasal congestion, or can manifest as asthma or eczema. Skin tests at your allergist's office are the best way to determine which pollens are triggering your child's allergic symptoms.

The best way to control a pollen allergy is to control one's exposure to pollen. That's easier said than done, of course; as parents, we relish few sights more than our child running around outside in the fresh air on a beautiful, breezy spring day. Outdoor pollen is simply out of our control, although you should know that pollen levels tend to be highest in the morning before 10 A.M. But we *can* control the

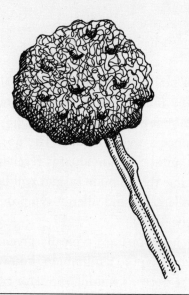

Molds reproduce by forming microscopic spores, which travel through the air. Proteins in the mold and spores cause allergic reactions in many children.

amount of pollen our children are exposed to indoors, which is where most children spend the majority of their time. Here are some basic guidelines for keeping as much pollen as possible outside, where it belongs.

- Keep windows closed during pollen season, and run air conditioners if necessary
- Remove shoes at the door
- Change your child's clothing as soon as he or she is indoors for the rest of the day
- Give your child a bath and shampoo immediately after he or she comes indoors, to remove pollen on skin and hair
- Don't dry bathing suits, towels, or other clothing outdoors, as these might become covered with pollen
- Don't do yardwork when your child is outdoors with you; any sort of vigorous digging, raking, mowing, or pruning can stir up pollen

IMMUNOTHERAPY

Some children with pollen and other seasonal allergies will benefit from immunotherapy (allergy shots). Immunotherapy introduces a small, controlled amount of allergen into the body at regularly timed intervals—usually once a week to start. The dose increases slightly with each injection, until the individual is receiving a full, optimum dose. Ideally, over time the immune system will become desensitized to the allergen or allergens, and allergy symptoms will decrease or disappear completely.

Immunotherapy injections are typically given with a very small needle, so discomfort is kept to a minimum. You will be asked to stay with your child in the doctor's waiting room for twenty to thirty minutes after the injection, in the unlikely event of an allergic reaction. You may also be asked to keep your child as quiet as possible for an hour or two before and an hour or two after the injection.

Immunotherapy requires a fairly lengthy commitment; it may take a year or more in order to experience significant relief from symptoms. But the experience of hundreds of thousands of children has proved that it can be very effective for those suffering from sensitivities to dust mites, tree and grass pollens, weed pollens, and mold. If your allergist suggests immunotherapy, rest assured that it is considered a very safe and very effective form of treatment.

Reading an ingredients label can make even the most erudite among us feel practically illiterate. What on Earth are all those bizarre items, and what are they doing in the food I'm about to give my precious child? The good news is that once you start reading labels, you find out both the good and the bad about the foods many of us have taken for granted. Carrageenan may have an exotic name, but it's really just a natural extract from seaweed. On the other hand, who ever knew how many places high-fructose corn syrup could show up?

This glossary was prepared by the Food Allergy Network and is included in its *Food Allergy News Cookbook*. FAN has graciously agreed to let me share it with all of you.

Agar-agar A complex carbohydrate extract from several varieties of red seaweed. It has the ability to swell and form a gel. It is used as a gelling agent in foods.

Albumins Natural components of animal products, egg albumin (ovalbumin) is found in the egg white, while lactalbumin is found in whey, the liquid part of milk. Albumins are used as additives in diet supplements, and as stabilizers, thickeners, and texturizers in a variety of foods. They are not safe for children allergic to eggs or milk.

Algae A group of plants that include seaweed and many single-cell marine and freshwater plants. This group includes some common food additives: agar-agar, alginates, and carrageenan.

Alginates Extracts from both red and brown seaweed, used as emulsifiers, to blend ingredients and prevent separation and as gels or thickeners.

BHA (butylated hydroxyanisole) and BHT (butylated hydroxytoluene) Synthetic compounds used as preservatives to prevent or delay the spoilage of fats, oils, and fat-containing foods.

Calcium peroxide Synthetic compound added to flours to ensure uniform quality. It also acts as a bleaching agent to extend the shelf life of flours.

Calcium phosphate, potassium phosphate, sodium phosphate Commercially prepared from phosphoric acid. Used as a flavoring agent and to prevent foods from separating. Found in many instant foods. Is also useful for varying acid or alkaline nature of food and as a nutritional supplement.

Calcium stearoyl-2-lactylate and sodium stearoyl-2-lactylate Produced by combining lactic acid and stearic acid, these act as dough conditioners to produce a more stable, durable dough. Also used as whipping agents for icings and as an emulsifier in coffee creamers and salad dressings.

Caramel Manufactured by the heating of various sugars to produce caramel flavoring or by heating the sugars along with an acid or alkaline salt to produce caramel color. The sugars that may be used in this process are dextrose, sucrose, molasses, malt syrup, and lactose. Caramel made from lactose would not be safe for children who are allergic to milk. When in doubt, avoid it. If you see caramel color listed on a product you would like to give your child, contact the manufacturer to verify the source of the caramel.

Carob A flavoring made from the pods of the carob tree, it tastes similar to chocolate but contains no caffeine. Carob is available in powder or in chips. If your child is allergic to milk, read the label to be sure that the carob chips are milk-free.

Carotene, beta-carotene A yellow-orange pigment that is found in fruits and vegetables. Carotene can be converted by the body to vitamin A. Is both a coloring agent and a nutritional supplement.

Carrageenan Also known as Irish moss, carrageenan is extracted from a variety of red algae. Like the alginates, it can be an emulsifier and a stabilizer to keep mixtures from separating, and a gelling and thickening agent.

Casein and caseinates Prepared from a process that uses skim milk to form a casein curd that is washed and dried. Caseinates are then produced by dissolving the casein in an alkaline solution that is sprayed or roller dried. Casein and caseinates are used as binders, extenders, clarifying agents, and dietary supplements. Because they are made from milk, they are not safe for milk-allergic children.

EDTA (ethylenediamine tetraacetic acid), calcium disodium EDTA, and disodium EDTA Chemical compounds that tightly bind to metals, such as copper and iron, can cause oxidation and rancidity, and change the flavor and texture of food. EDTA prevents these reactions and improves stability and shelf life of foods.

Gluten A mixture of proteins present in wheat flour, obtained as an extremely sticky, yellowish gray mass by making a dough and then washing out the starch. Gluten consists almost entirely of two proteins, gliadin and glutelin, the exact proportions of which depend on the variety of wheat. Gluten contributes to the porous and spongy structure of bread. Children with celiac sprue must avoid eating gluten-containing products.

Gum arabic, acacia A gum obtained from a number of species of acacia, a Middle Eastern tree. Gum arabic is a complex carbohydrate that dissolves in water, making it useful as a food additive. It is used as a blender, a thickener, and to improve texture.

Hydrolyzed casein Made from casein, a milk protein, that has been treated with enzymes. Not safe for milk-allergic children.

Hydrolyzed plant protein (HPP) and hydrolyzed vegetable protein (HVP) Produced by the hydrolysis of soybean and peanut meals, or from protein recovered from the wet milling of grains. Although soybeans are the primary source of most HPP and HVP, if your child is allergic to peanuts you should avoid this substance or contact the manufacturer to find out if it's peanut- or soybean-derived.

Lactic acid Produced in commercial foods either by chemical synthesis or from bacterial fermentation of a carbohydrate such as corn sugar.

Lecithin A complex mixture of fatty substances derived primarily from the processing of soybeans but also from corn and eggs. The main components of lecithin are choline, phosphoric acid, glycerin, and fatty acids. Choline is chemically synthesized for use as a food additive. Glycerin is an alcohol that is a component of all fats. Most companies clearly label when egg lecithin is used, but if your child is severely egg-allergic or you have any doubts about the ingredients, you should contact the manufacturer. Lecithin is used as an emulsifier, a stabilizer, and an antioxidant.

Locust bean gum, also known as carob bean gum or carob seed gum Extracted from the seed of a carob tree, this gum is used as a blender, a stabilizer, a binder, and to improve the texture of foods.

Malt Produced from germinated barley, malt syrup is a thick concentrate extracted from malt with water. Dried malt extract, a powder, is produced by drying the syrup. It is used to flavor foods and to make breads, beer, and whiskey.

Pareve When *pareve* is printed on a food label, it means the product was prepared without either meat or milk products. Hence, it is permissible to eat this product with either meat or dairy dishes in accordance with Jewish dietary laws. This symbol is useful for people on milk-restricted diets. *However*, a label marked *pareve* is not a guarantee that absolutely no milk protein whatsoever exists in the food. Tiny amounts of milk protein—a small amount of powdered milk, for instance, that is airborne in the same factory where the pareve product is being manufactured—may be present in the product. People who are severely allergic to milk should not rely on the pareve symbol alone when determining if a food is safe to eat.

Propionic acid, calcium propionate, and sodium propionate Produced by chemical synthesis for the food industry to inhibit mold growth and to preserve foods.

Protein hydrolysates Mixtures of amino acids naturally found in foods; amino acids are the primary components of proteins. They are extracted from foods by various chemical and manufacturing processes.

Sorbitan derivatives: polysorbate 60, 65, 80 and sorbitan monostearate Produced by chemically dehydrating sorbitol, a simple sugar-alcohol, these additives are used as emulsifiers.

Starch, gelatinized starch, modified starch Obtained from a variety of foods, including tapioca, potatoes, corn, wheat, and rice, food starch is produced by steeping and grinding the seed or tuber of the plant to make a slurry. Sulfur dioxide is then added to separate the protein from the starch. These resulting food starches are used as thickening and gelling agents.

Tapioca A beady starch derived from the root of the tropical cassava plant. Used for puddings and as a thickening agent in cooking.

Tofu A white, easily digestible curd made from cooked soybeans. High in protein, tofu contains no cholesterol and readily accepts flavors from the foods it is cooked with. Available in soft (silken) and firm varieties, tofu must be avoided by people allergic to soy.

Whey The liquid portion of milk that remains after the casein has been removed. It is used in many foods as a source of protein and minerals but should be avoided by people allergic to milk.

Copyright © by the Food Allergy Network. Reprinted by permission of the Food Allergy Network.

APPENDIX B:
FOOD MANUFACTURERS

The following is a basic list of major food manufacturers and their consumer information lines. It has been my experience that these companies are very helpful and cooperative in dealing with food-allergy issues.

Beech-Nut
Box 618
St. Louis, MO 63188
(800) 523-6633

Best Foods Baking Group
(Arnold, Brownberry, Thomas)
100 Passaic Avenue
Fairfield, NJ 07004
(800) 356-3314

Betty Crocker
(A division of General Mills)
Box 113
Minneapolis, MN 55440
Cereal: (800) 328-1144
Desserts and convenience foods:
(800) 328-6787
Snacks: (800) 231-0308

Borden
180 East Broad Street
Columbus, OH 43215
(614) 225-4511

Campbell Soup Company
(Campbell, Franco-American, V-8,
Swanson, Prego, Pepperidge Farm,
Vlasic, Marie's, Mrs. Paul's, Godiva)
1 Campbell Place
Camden, NJ 08103
(800) 770-5858 or (800) 257-8443

Dannon Co., Inc.
P.O. Box 44235
Jacksonville, FL 32231
(800) 321-2174

Gerber Foods
Gerber Products
Fremont, MI 49413
(800) 4-GERBER

Healthy Choice
ConAgra Frozen Foods
Box 3768
Omaha, NE 68103
(800) 323-9980

H. J. Heinz
1062 Progress Street
Pittsburgh, PA 15212
(412) 237-5740
Baby food: (800) 872-2229

Heinz Frozen Foods Company
 (formerly Ore-Ida Foods)
Box 10
Boise, ID 83707
(208) 383-6800

Hershey Foods
100 Crystal A Drive
Hershey, PA 17033
(800) 468-1714

Kellogg Company
Box CAMB
Battle Creek, MI 49016
(800) 962-1718

Kraft/General Foods
Glenview, IL 60025
(800) 634-1984
Cereal: (800) 431-POST

Nabisco Foods
East Hanover, NJ 07936
(800) 932-7800

Pillsbury
Box 550
Minneapolis, MN 55440
(800) 767-4466

Quaker Oats Company
P.O. Box 049003
Chicago, IL 60604
(800) 494-7843

Sara Lee Bakery Products
224 South Michigan Avenue
Chicago, IL 60604
(800) 323-7117

CHAIN RESTAURANTS AND FRANCHISES

In recent years, many national restaurant chains and franchises have begun making ingredients lists available to the public. Some fast-food restaurants even display these lists on a poster or have them available behind the counter. Other restaurants can send or fax you their lists. Make sure they are up-to-date, as menus and the ingredients used may change. If you are a member of the Food Allergy Network (FAN), you will receive advance warning regarding ingredient changes in the menus of several national restaurant chains and franchises.

While the degree of allergy awareness may vary greatly from location to location, most are at least aware of the problems and are willing to work with you. When you are dealing with a national chain, bear in mind that different regions may have the flexibility to vary their ingredients slightly. It's always best to consult the ingredients list first, then inquire at your local outlet.

Arby's
Box 407008
Ft. Lauderdale, FL 33340
(800) 487-2729

Boston Market
1804 Centre Point Drive
P.O. Box 3117
Naperville, IL 60566
(800) 365-7000

Burger King
17777 Old Cutler Road
Miami, FL 33157
(305) 378-3535

Carvel Corporation
Ft. Lauderdale, FL 33340
(800) 322-4848

Denny's
203 East Main Street
Spartanburg, SC 29319
(800) 733-6697

Friendly's
1855 Boston Road
Wilbraham, MA 01095
(413) 543-2400

International House of Pancakes
525 North Brand Boulevard
Glendale, CA 91203
(800) 241-4467

KFC/Kentucky Fried Chicken
KFC Inc.
P.O. Box 32070
Louisville, KY 40232
(800) CALL KFC

McDonald's Corporation
One Kroc Drive
Oak Brook, IL 60521

Subway
325 Bic Drive
Milford, CT 06460
(800) 888-4848

Taco Bell
1701 Von Karman Avenue
Irvine, CA 92714
(800) TAC-OBEL

Wendy's
4288 West Dublin Gramville Road
Dublin, OH 43017
(800) 443-7266

ACKNOWLEDGMENTS

I am honored to have had the chance to work with Hugh A. Sampson, M.D., and Sally Noone, R.N., of the Elliot and Roslyn Jaffe Institute for Food Allergy at Mount Sinai Medical Center. Thank you both for your generosity, good humor, priceless information, patience, and accessibility. You are my heroes.

A writer could not have better professional partners than Maryanne Scott, M.D., and Elinor Greenberg, Ph.D. You talked, I learned; we all laughed a lot. It doesn't get much better than that.

A special thank you to David and Helen Jaffe, who opened all the doors, seemed to divine what I needed before I even asked, and were always available yet never once asked to look at the manuscript. Your faith in this project made every day of work a joy. Thank you to Aimie Rappoport, director of the Food Allergy Initiative, for your warmth and cooperation every step of the way.

To Anne Munoz-Furlong, founder and president of the Food Allergy Network, my lifelong gratitude. Your work makes life better for tens of thousands each day, but you always manage to keep it one-on-one.

I am lucky to have worked with two people who taught me what great good fun it is to work hard and write well: Mark Peel and Lewis M. Smith,

Jr. You are still the coaches I turn to in my head when it isn't coming out quite right.

I would like to thank my husband, David, for his noble technical achievements in the service of getting this book to the publisher, including one memorable all-nighter; my son Dylan, for being such an understanding and protective big brother; my parents, Annette and Marvin Krauss, and Stephen Schapiro, who were possibly even more excited about this project than I was; and Edwin and Virginia Barber, who since the first day we met have meant the world to me.

Thank you to my special friends who listened, offered endless feedback, and cheered me on at every opportunity, especially:

Tracey Bloom
Karin Fraade
Linda Gray
Beth Hapke, M.D.
Bobbie Heibeck
Stacy Kamisar
Shirley Matthews
Lisa Pesco
Ellyn Weitzman

Thank you to Heather Klein, Susan Weeks, Audrey Ludemann, Colleen O'Neill, Debbie Magrone, Linda Feldstein, and Gina DeMarco for being the kind of educators who inspire complete confidence not only in a child's learning but in his safety as well. And a special thank you to Dr. Janet Shaner, Dr. Len Tomasello, Nurse Cathy Nucera, and the staff of Hurlbutt Elementary School, who have truly risen to the occasion of protecting all food-allergic students.

Finally, thank you to my editor Deb Brody, who raised her hand first when this project was proposed, and who has led it forward with matter-of-fact good sense, good cheer, and decisiveness. As happy as I was to hand in the manuscript, I was sorry for the process to end.

INDEX

ABOUT THE AUTHOR

Marianne Barber, the mother of a food-allergic child, is an award-winning copywriter and a founding member of the Connecticut chapter of the Food Allergy Initiative (FAI). This nonprofit group works closely with the Food Allergy Network (FAN) to increase public awareness of food-allergy issues, raise funds for research, and help families and communities create a safer environment for all food-allergic individuals. Born and raised in New York, she attended the Fiorello H. LaGuardia High School of Music and the Performing Arts, and later Colgate University. Marianne now lives with her husband, David, and sons, Dylan and Lucas, in Weston, Connecticut.